COMPLICATIONS OF LASER SURGERY
OF THE HEAD AND NECK

Complications of Laser Surgery of the Head and Neck

Marvin P. Fried, M.D.
Associate Professor of Otolaryngology
Harvard Medical School
Boston, Massachusetts

James H. Kelly, M.D.
Associate Professor of Otolaryngology-
Head and Neck Surgery
The Johns Hopkins Medical School
Baltimore, Maryland

Marshall Strome, M.D.
Associate Professor of Otolaryngology
Harvard Medical School
Boston, Massachusetts

YEAR BOOK MEDICAL PUBLISHERS, INC.
CHICAGO • LONDON

1 2 3 4 5 6 7 8 9 0 C Y 8 9 8 8 8 7 8 6

Library of Congress Cataloging-in-Publication Data

Complications of laser surgery of the head and neck.

Includes bibliographies and index.
1. Head—Surgery—Complications and sequelae.
2. Neck—Surgery—Complications and sequelae.
3. Lasers in surgery—Complications and sequelae.
4. Lasers in surgery—Safety measures. I. Fried, Marvin P. II. Kelly, James H. III. Strome, Marshall, 1940- . [DNLM: 1. Head—surgery. 2. Lasers—adverse effects. 3. Lasers—therapeutic use. 4. Neck—surgery. 5. Postoperative Complications. WE 705 C7395]
RD521.C654 1986 617′.5101 85-29539
ISBN 0-8151-3291-3

Sponsoring Editor: David K. Marshall
Manager, Copyediting Services: Frances M. Perveiler
Production Project Manager: Max Perez
Proofroom Supervisor: Shirley E. Taylor

To my wife, Rita, and my exciting daughters, Karen and Jaimie, for their support, understanding, and love. MPF

To Jane, with love. JHK

To Deena, Scott, and Randy, a greater blessing life cannot bestow. MS

Contributors

MARVIN P. FRIED, M.D.
Associate Professor of Otolaryngology
Harvard Medical School
Boston, Massachusetts

GERALD B. HEALY, M.D.
Professor of Otolaryngology
Boston University School of Medicine
Associate Professor of Otolaryngology
Harvard Medical School
Boston, Massachusetts

JAMES H. KELLY, M.D.
Associate Professor of Otolaryngology-Head and Neck Surgery
The Johns Hopkins Medical School
Baltimore, Maryland

BRENDA J. MCKONLY, R.N.
Head Nurse, Operating Room
Beth Israel Hospital
Boston, Massachusetts

JOEL M. NOE, M.D., F.A.C.S., P.C.
Assistant Professor of Plastic and Reconstructive Surgery
Harvard Medical School
Boston, Massachusetts

EDWARD V. NORTON, M.D.
Legal Research Associate
Department of Anesthesiology
University of Michigan Medical Center
Ann Arbor, Michigan

MARTIN L. NORTON, M.D., J.D.
Professor of Anesthesiology of Counsel
University of Michigan School of Medicine
Ann Arbor, Michigan

ROBERT H. OSSOFF, D.M.D., M.D.
Associate Professor of Otolaryngology-Head and Neck Surgery
Northwestern University Medical School
Head, Division of Otolaryngology-Head and Neck Surgery
Evanston Hospital
Evanston, Illinois

CAROL A. RICHARD, R.N.
Head Nurse, Operating Room
Brigham and Women's Hospital
Boston, Massachusetts

R. JAMES ROCKWELL, JR., M.SC.
President, Rockwell Associates, Inc.
Cincinnati, Ohio

STANLEY M. SHAPSHAY, M.D., F.A.C.S.
Assistant Professor of Otolaryngology-Head and Neck Surgery
Chairman, Department of Otolaryngology-Head and Neck Surgery
Boston University School of Medicine
Director of Eleanor Naylor Dana Laser Research Laboratory
Boston, Massachusetts

MARSHALL STROME, M.D.
Associate Professor of Otolaryngology
Harvard Medical School
Boston, Massachusetts

DAVID M. VERNICK, M.D.
Instructor in Otolaryngology
Harvard Medical School
Boston, Massachusetts

Preface

The surgical laser has evolved from early bulky, complicated, and cumbersome machines to the relatively easy-to-set-up models of today. In most cases, using a surgical laser has become less complicated than using a video game. Thus, it is easy to forget that the laser is a powerful (and potentially dangerous) surgical instrument. Although newer models are safer and more reliable than the earlier lasers, errors in judgment and careless use will still produce injuries. In fact, because they are relatively easy to use, constant attention by all personnel involved with the laser must be exhibited to reduce injuries. Moreover, the use of the surgical laser has grown dramatically over the past decade. Not only has the number of lasers (and hospitals using them) increased, but, similarly, the types of surgery. An increasing case load and number of practitioners potentiates a heightened number of complications.

It is the purpose of this book to provide an overview of potential safety hazards and to delineate ways to reduce them. Despite all precautions, injuries will result; therefore methods to minimize and treat these injuries are also included. We have attempted to approach this subject from the various types of lasers (CO_2, argon, Nd:YAG), and surgical procedures, as well as from the perspectives of each of the hospital personnel that are involved in the use of the laser (surgeon, anesthesiologist, nurse). Finally, because injuries will occur, we have included a chapter delineating legal liabilities.

The readers of this book will notice a certain amount of repetitiveness in the chapters, particularly in regard to safety precautions. Because of the philosophy to approach the same occurrence from a variety of viewpoints, this repetition is inevitable, but will serve to stress important safety considerations and the treatment of complications.

The authors recognize that further advances in laser technology may solve many of the problems that are mentioned here. This technology advance will also inevitably produce problems that cannot be anticipated.

It is the hope of the editors that this book can be used as a guide to stimulate an organized approach to safety with regard to the surgical laser. The authors realize that this book cannot take the place of a carefully designed educational program involving all personnel. Constant updating of this education is mandatory as new advances in laser technology occur.

Marvin P. Fried, M.D.
James H. Kelly, M.D.
Marshall Strome, M.D.

Contents

watt CO_2 lasers are currently undergoing trials for "welding" small vessels, anastomosing nerves, eradicating residual epithelial deposits in the mastoid, and selectively destroying components of the vestibular system. At this time, only the physician's imagination seems to be the limitation for future applicability.

BIBLIOGRAPHY

1. Fuller T.A.: The physics of surgical lasers. *Lasers Surg. Med.* 1:5–14, 1980.
2. Toty L., Personne C., Colchen A., et al.: Bronchoscopic management of tracheal lesions using the neodynium yttrium aluminum garnet laser. *Thorax* 36:175–178, 1981.
3. Clark W.C., Robertson J.H., Gardner G.: Selective absorption and control of thermal effects: A comparison of the laser systems used in otology and neurotology. *Otolaryngol. Head Neck Surg.* 92:75–79, 1984.

2 Laser Concepts, Tissue Interactions, and Safety Practices

R. James Rockwell, Jr., M.Sc.

THE IMPORTANCE OF LASER CONCEPTS: AN OVERVIEW

The field of laser surgery has advanced rapidly in the past decade. This is not at all surprising when one considers the many advantages that lasers offer to surgeons. The basic medical advantages of laser surgery include noncontact, dry field, highly sterile, very localized operations with a clear field of view. The basic laser-tissue interaction can aid in prompt healing by minimizing tissue swelling and scarring. It should be understood, however, that lasers do emit intense, coherent electromagnetic radiation (EMR) with the potential for causing damage to the skin and eye of humans.

FUNDAMENTALS AND CHARACTERISTICS OF LASERS

Fundamentals

The term *laser* is an acronym. It stands for *l*ight *a*mplification by *s*timulated *e*mission of *r*adiation. Thus the laser is a device that produces and amplifies light. The mechanism by which this is accomplished, stimulated emission, was first postulated by Einstein in 1917. The light that the laser produces is unique, for it is characterized by properties that are very desirable, but almost impossible to obtain by any means other than the laser.

To gain a better understanding of the laser and what it can do, a review of some of the phenomena involved in laser action starting with the nature of light itself will be discussed.

Electromagnetic Spectrum

Light is a form of electromagnetic energy. It occupies that portion of the electromagnetic spectrum with which humans first dealt because it was visible to the human eye. Originally, the term *light* included only the visible frequencies. In about 1800, however, the British-German astronomer W. Herschel placed a thermometer just beyond the blue portion of a light spectrum produced by passing sunlight through a prism and found that the temperature was raised. Later, invisible light was also found on the other end of the visible spectrum (beyond visible red light). Thus it was that frequencies *outside* the visible range were lumped with the visible frequencies under the term *light.*

Later, when x-rays, radiowaves, and other discoveries were made, light was found to be part of a total spectrum of EMRs. The distinction between the various radiations is the frequency of the oscillation of the electric (and/or magnetic) fields of which the light is comprised. "Light" is considered to be that portion of the electromagnetic spectrum having wavelengths between 100 and 10,000 nm (nm = 10^{-9} m). The various divisions of the complete electromagnetic spectrum are shown in Figure 2–1.

From a classical viewpoint, light simultaneously displays two seemingly contradictory properties: (1) waves that propagate through space and (2) "particles" that have a discrete energy and momentum called photons.

Each of these properties is important to the complete understanding of the behavior of all EMRs. Both properties are combined in the current concept of light as described in modern physics by quantum mechanics.

Frequently, as an aid in visualizing wave behavior, light is said to move in much the same fashion as waves on a body of water. While this is not entirely true, certain characteristics are common to both types of wave motions.

The fact that a definite energy is associated with the radiation is often considered a particle-like property. It is therefore difficult to visualize EMRs as continuous waves, propagating continuously through space. One means of partially relieving this conceptual difficulty is thinking of the radiations as consisting of a limited "wave pocket" which is called a "photon." The energy packet, or photon (Figure 2–2), is thought to move through space, thus satisfying a human need to visualize that which one cannot truly visualize.

Electron Energy Levels

Light can be produced by atomic processes, and it is these processes that are responsible for the generation of laser light. Let's look first at atomic

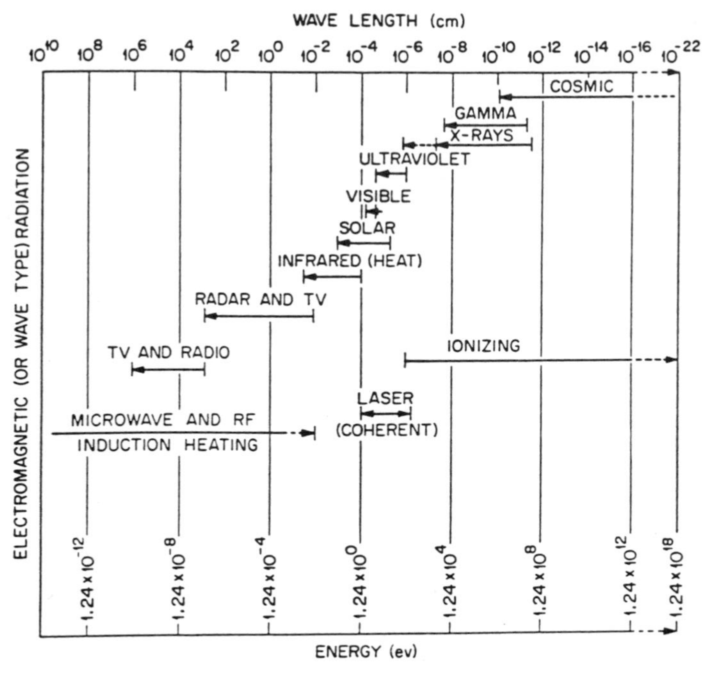

Fig 2–1. The electromagnetic spectrum.

energy levels and then see how changes in these energy levels can lead to the production of laser light.

A number of simplifications will be made regarding the concept of the atom. We can assume, for purposes of this discussion, that an atom consists of a small dense nucleus and one or more electrons in motion about the nucleus.

The relationship between the electrons and the nucleus is described in terms of energy levels. Quantum mechanics predicts that these energy levels are discrete. A simplified energy level diagram as shown in Figure 2–3 makes it easy to visualize these discrete energy levels.

Radiative Transitions

The electrons normally occupy the lowest available energy levels. When this is the case, the atom is said to be in its *ground state.* However, electrons can occupy higher energy levels, leaving some of the lower energy states vacant or sparsely populated.

One way that electrons can change from one energy state to another is by the *absorption* or *emission* of a photon. One of the ways in which an atom can change its energy state is through what is called a radiative transition.

There are three types of radiative transitions. Two of these, *absorption* and *spontaneous emission,* are quite familiar, but the third, *stimulated emission* is relatively unfamiliar. It is this third type of radiative transition that forms the basis for the laser action. Each form of transition is described below.

Absorption.—An electron can absorb energy from a variety of external sources. From the point of view of laser action, two methods of supplying energy to the electrons are of prime importance. The first of these is the transfer of all the energy of a photon directly to an orbital electron. The increase in the energy of the electron causes it to "jump" to a higher energy level; the atom is then said to be in an "excited" state. It is important to note that an electron can accept only the precise amount of energy that is needed to move it from one allowable energy level to another. Only photons of the *exact energy* acceptable to the electron can be absorbed. Photons of slightly more (or slightly less) energy will *not* be absorbed.

Another means often used to excite electrons is an electrical discharge. In this technique, the energy is supplied by collisions with electrons that have been accelerated by an electric field. The result of either type of excitation is that through the absorption of energy, an electron has been placed in a higher energy level than it originally resided. As a result, the atom of which it is part is said to be "excited."

Spontaneous Emission.—The nature of all matter is such that atomic and molecular structures tend to exist in the lowest energy state possible. Thus, an excited electron in a higher energy level will soon attempt to "de-

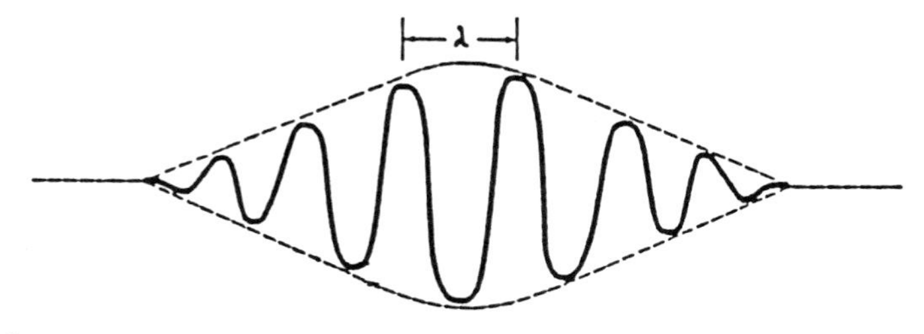

Fig 2–2. Representation of a photon combining the concept of wave-like properties together with a finite energy packet. (From Rockwell R.J.: *Laser Safety in Surgery and Medicine.* Cincinnati, Ohio, Rockwell Associates, Inc., 1985. Reproduced by permission.)

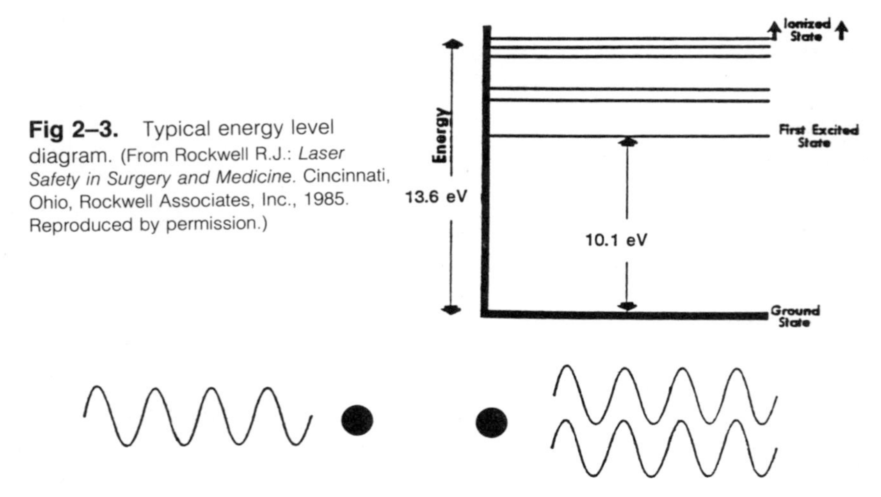

Fig 2–3. Typical energy level diagram. (From Rockwell R.J.: *Laser Safety in Surgery and Medicine*. Cincinnati, Ohio, Rockwell Associates, Inc., 1985. Reproduced by permission.)

Fig 2–4. Apparent photon multiplication by stimulated emission. (From Rockwell R.J.: *Laser Safety in Surgery and Medicine*. Cincinnati, Ohio, Rockwell Associates, Inc., 1985. Reproduced by permission.)

excite" itself by any of several means. Some of the energy may be converted to heat. Another means of de-excitation is the spontaneous emission of a photon. The photon released by an atom as it is de-excited will have a total energy exactly equal to the difference in energy between the excited and lower energy levels. This release of a photon is called spontaneous emission. One example of spontaneous emission is the common neon sign. Atoms of neon are excited by an electrical discharge through the tube. They de-excite themselves by spontaneously emitting photons of visible light. Note that the exciting force is not of a unique energy, so that the electrons may be excited to any one of several energy levels.

Now let us look at the third, and probably the least familiar, type of radiative transition.

Stimulated Emission.—In 1917, Einstein postulated that a photon released from an excited atom could, on interacting with a second, similarly excited atom, trigger the second atom into de-exciting itself with the release of a photon. The photon released by the second atom would be identical in frequency, energy, direction, and phase with the triggering photon, *and* the triggering photon would continue on its way, unchanged. Where there was one photon now there are two. These two photons could then proceed to trigger more through the process of stimulated emission, as depicted in Figure 2–4.

If an appropriate medium contains a great many excited atoms and de-excitation occurs, *only* by spontaneous emission, the light output will be random and approximately equal in all directions.

The process of stimulated emission, however, can cause an amplification of the number of photons traveling in a particular direction—a photon cascade if you will. A preferential direction is established by placing mirrors at the ends of an optical cavity, as shown in Figure 2–5. Thus, the number of photons traveling along the axis of the two mirrors increased greatly and "*l*ight *a*mplification by the *s*timulated *e*mission of *r*adiation" occurs. A LASER beam is, therefore, created.

Population Inversion

Practically speaking, the process of stimulated emission will not produce a very efficient or even noticeable amplification of light unless a condition called "population inversion" occurs. If only two of several million atoms are in an excited state, the changes of stimulated emission occurring are infinitely small. The greater the percentage of atoms in an excited state, the greater the probability of stimulated emission. In the normal state of matter as shown in Figure 2–6, the population of electrons will be such that most of the electrons reside in the ground or lowest energy levels, leaving the upper levels somewhat depopulated. When electrons are excited and fill these upper levels to the extent that there are more atoms excited than not excited, the population is said to be *inverted*.

Laser Components

A generalized laser consists of a lasting medium, a "pumping" system, and an optical cavity. The laser material must have a metastable state in which

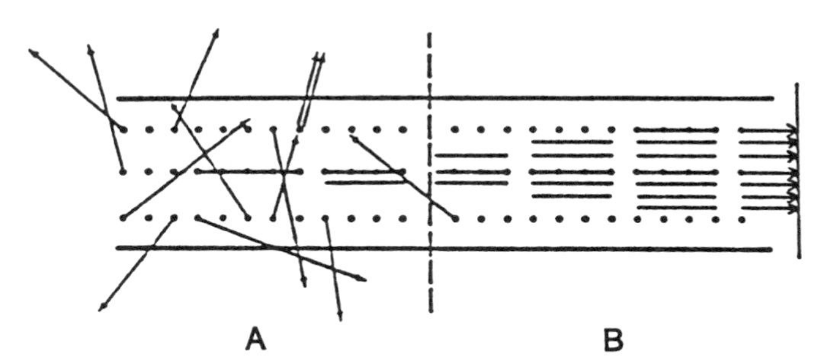

Fig 2–5. Photon cascade that occurs in the stimulated emission process. (From Rockwell R.J.: *Laser Safety in Surgery and Medicine*. Cincinnati, Ohio, Rockwell Associates, Inc., 1985. Reproduced by permission.)

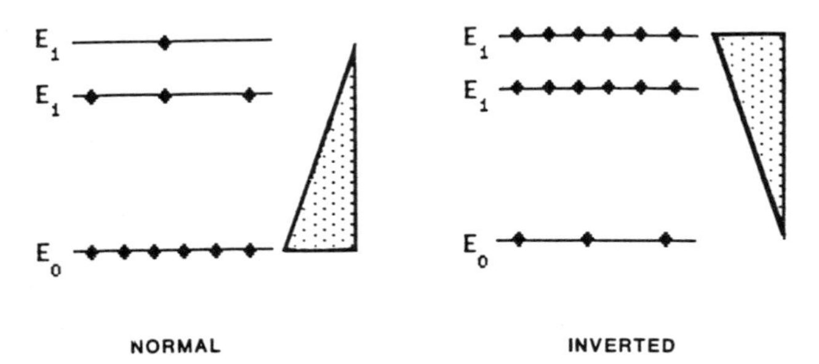

Fig 2–6. Comparison between normal and inverted population distribution. (From Rockwell R.J.: *Laser Safety in Surgery and Medicine*. Cincinnati, Ohio, Rockwell Associates, Inc., 1985. Reproduced by permission.)

the atoms or molecules can be trapped after receiving energy from the pumping system. Each of these laser components are discussed below.

Pumping Systems.—The pumping system imparts energy to the atoms or molecules of the lasting medium, enabling them to be raised to an excited "metastable state" creating a population inversion.

Optical pumping uses photons provided by a source such as Xenon gas flash tube or another laser to transfer energy to the lasing material. The optical source must provide photons that correspond to the allowed transition levels of the lasing material.

Collision pumping relies on the transfer of energy to the lasing material by collision with the atoms (or molecules) of the lasing material. Again, energies that correspond to the allowed transitions must be provided.

Chemical pumping systems use the binding energy released in chemical reactions to raise the lasing material to the metastable state.

Optical Cavity.—An optical cavity is required to provide the amplification desired in the laser and to select the photons that are traveling in the desired direction. As the first atom or molecule in the metastable state of the inverted population decays, it triggers via stimulated emission, the decay of another atom or molecule in the metastable state. If the photons are traveling in a direction that leads to the walls of the lasing material, which is usually in the form of a rod or tube, they are lost and the amplification process terminates. They may actually be reflected at the wall of the rod or tube, but sooner or later they will be lost in the system and will not contribute to the beam.

If, on the other hand, one of the decaying atoms or molecules releases a photon parallel to the axis of the lasing material, it can trigger the emission of another photon and both will be reflected by the mirror on the end of the lasing rod or tube. The reflected photons then pass back through the material triggering further emissions along exactly the same path, which are reflected by the mirrors on the ends of the lasing material. As this amplification process continues, a portion of the radiation will always escape through the partially reflecting mirror. In this way, a narrow concentrated beam of coherent light is formed.

The mirrors on the laser optical cavity must be precisely aligned for light beams parallel to the axis. The optical cavity itself, i.e., the lasing medium material must not be a stronger absorber of the light energy.

Lasing Media

Lasers are commonly designated by the type of lasing material employed. There are four types: solid state, gas, dye, and semiconductor. The characteristics of each type will be described.

Solid State Lasers.—Solid state lasers employ a lasing material distributed in a solid matrix. One example is the ruby laser, using a precise amount of chromium impurity distributed uniformly in a rod of crystalline aluminum oxide. The laser output is generated primarily at a wavelength of 694.3 nm, which is deep red. Another solid state laser (now gaining expanded use as a surgery laser) is the Neodymium:YAG (Nd:YAG) laser. The abbreviation YAG is for the crystal *y*ttrium *a*luminium *g*arnet, which serves as the host for the neodymium ions. This laser emits an infrared beam at a wavelength of 1.064 μm ($\mu m = 10^{-6}$ m).

Gas Lasers.—Gas lasers use a gas or a mixture of gases within a tube. The most common gas laser is the helium-neon (He-Ne), with a primary output of 632.8 nm, which is a visible red. It was first developed in 1961 and has proved to be the forerunner of a whole family of gas lasers. All gas lasers are quite similar in construction and behavior. The CO_2 gas laser radiates at 10.6 μm in the far-infrared spectrum. Argon and krypton gas lasers, with multiple frequency emissions in the visible spectra, are becoming quite common for use in surgery and ophthalmology—particularly when blue or green light is desired. The principal emission wavelengths of an argon laser are 488 and 514 nm.

Dye Lasers.—The laser medium in dye lasers is usually a complex organic dye in liquid solution or suspension. The most striking feature of these lasers is their "tunability." Proper choice of the dye and its concentration allows the production of laser light over a broad range of wavelengths in or near the visible spectrum. Dye lasers commonly employ optical pumping, although some types have used chemical reaction pumping. The most commonly used dye is Rhodamine 6G, which provides tunability over a 200-nm bandwidth in the red portion of the spectrum.

Semiconductor Lasers.—Semiconductor (diode) lasers are not to be confused with solid state lasers. Semiconductor devices consist of two layers of semiconductor material sandwiched together. These lasers are generally very *small* physically, and individually of low power. However, they may be made into larger arrays. The most common diode laser is the Gallium Arsenide diode laser, with a central emission of 840 nm.

Modes of Operation

The different modes of operation of a laser are distinguished by the rate at which energy is delivered.

Continuous Wave.—In a continuously radiating laser, the beam power is constant with time.

Repetitively Pulsed or Scanning.—This operational mode is capable of pulse rates that may range from 10 to 1,000 pulses per second. Some systems employ optical scanning systems to produce the repetitively pulsed output.

Normal Pulse Mode.—In general, lasers operating in a normal pulse mode have pulse durations of a few hundred microseconds to a few milliseconds. This mode of operation is sometimes referred to as long pulse or pulsed.

Q-Switched.—An intracavity delay allows the laser media to store a maximum of potential energy. Then, under optimum gain conditions, emission occurs in single pulses of 10^{-8} second time domain with very high peak pulse powers.

Mode Locked.—The resonant modes of the optical cavity effect the characteristics of the output beam. The effect can vary from small transient effects to large fluctuations in the beam intensity over time.

When the phases of different frequency modes are synchronized, i.e., "locked together," the different modes will interfere with one another to generate a beat effect. The result will be a laser output that is observed as regularly spaced pulsations. Lasers operating in this mode-locked fashion usually produce trains of pulses, each having a duration of a few picoseconds (ps: 10^{-12} sec) to a few nanoseconds. A mode-locked laser can deliver extremely high peak power pulses. If pulse energies are maintained equal, the mode locked operation will produce significantly higher peak power than the same laser operating in the Q-switched mode.

CHARACTERISTICS

The following properties are common to the beams emitted from all laser types and are the factors which, when combined together, distinguish laser outputs from other sources of electromagnetic radiation:

1. A nearly single frequency operation of low bandwidth (i.e., an almost pure monochromatic light beam).

2. Emission of a nearly parallel beam with well-defined wavefronts in a Gaussian ("bell-shaped") distribution.

3. A beam of enormous intensity.

4. A beam that maintains a high degree of temporal and spatial coherence.

5. A beam that is, in many laser devices, highly plane polarized.

6. A beam with enormous electromagnetic field strengths.

Each of the above listed characteristics of a laser beam are briefly reviewed in the following sections.

Single Frequency Operation (Monochromaticity).—The frequency of any electromagnetic wave relates to the number of cycles the electric or magnetic field undergoes each second. The ideal laser will be a completely coherent, monochromatic wave oscillating exactly at a constant frequency. Most laser systems display a multifrequency characteristic. This frequency spread is, however, very narrow when compared with the average laser frequency. In most lasers, the frequency spread is solely dependent on the quantum transition characteristics of the active media and the geometry of the resonant cavity.

In this sense, the laser media may be considered as a high number of isolated light generators placed between two mirrors. The electromagnetic field developed between the mirrors may be regarded as a superposition of plane waves at each of the slightly different frequencies that the laser media generates and allows to oscillate. These different frequencies are termed the *modes* of the laser resonator and relate to the various electromagnetic field configurations that can exist between the two mirrors.

The lowest order axial mode is designated as the TEM_{00} mode and is shown in the left-hand part of Figure 2–7. This mode has the lowest diffraction losses and consequently will often be the predominant mode of oscillation. For each transverse mode, there will be many longitudinal modes that can oscillate; hence the output of the multimode laser will actually contain a superposition of plane waves oscillating at many discrete frequencies. However, as previously mentioned, this frequency spread will be very small.

For most cases, the average wavelength at which the laser oscillates is sufficient to describe the operation. If more precision is needed, then the frequency spread or bandwidth is given. Depending on the type of laser, bandwidths range typically from 10^{-4} to 10^{-9} times the average frequency of the laser, although bandwidths as low as 0.1 Hz have been reported for stabilized gas lasers.

Gaussian Distribution of Beam.—The laser's intensity profile across a TEM_{00} beam will be in the form of a bell-shaped or Gaussian distribution, as shown in Figure 2–8. The decrease in intensity near the edge of the beam is the result of diffraction effects produced at the edge of the laser beam. Departure from the Gaussian type distribution arises when independent oscillation occurs within the resonator at one of the higher order modes. For example, gas lasers may be designed to have sufficient gain to support simultaneous oscillation in many different transverse modes. Mode selection may often be accomplished by slight adjustment of the mirror alignments.

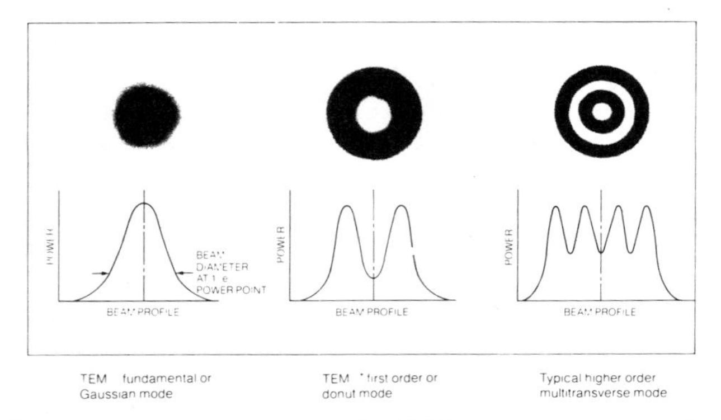

Fig 2–7. Transverse electromagnetic mode (TEM) patterns. Note complex spatial distributions of the higher order mode patterns. (From Rockwell R.J.: *Laser Safety in Surgery and Medicine.* Cincinnati, Ohio, Rockwell Associates, Inc., 1985. Reproduced by permission.)

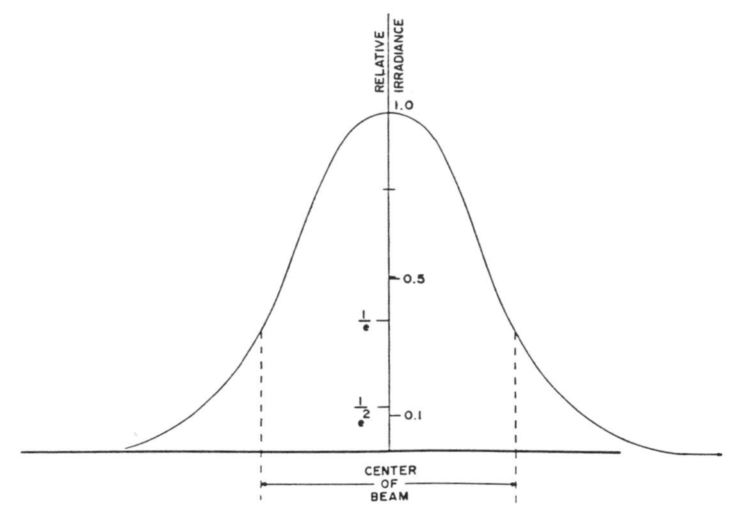

Fig 2–8. Gaussian beam distribution. (From Rockwell R.J.: *Laser Safety in Surgery and Medicine.* Cincinnati, Ohio, Rockwell Associates, Inc., 1985. Reproduced by permission.)

With this technique, one can observe the different complex intensity distributions of each mode. The lowest order TEM_{00} mode with the nearly Gaussian intensity distribution has the lowest cavity losses and hence will generally be the dominant mode of oscillation.

Optically pumped solid-state lasers—such as the normal mode ruby or Nd:YAG laser—usually display a randomly varying mode output. Thermal gradients in the optical media (i.e., the crystal) caused by nonuniform absorption of the pump light give rise to lens effects in the crystal that change during the pumping cycle. The result is a sporadic switching of transverse modes during the laser pulse. The time average is generally a bell-shaped distribution that is dependent on the optimal purity of the laser crystal, the pumping scheme, and the level at which the system is operated above the lasing threshold.

Some pumping schemes can produce pronounced "hot spots" in the intensity distributions. For long-range transmission, atmospheric effects can also produce large scale intensity variations over localized regions of the beam. Such nonuniformities in distribution make it difficult to specify the cross-sectional area of the beam. As a result, an average value of beam radius must be chosen.

The beam from an ideal laser, i.e., a laser that emits a coherent wave, can be considered to emit a diffraction-limited beam. In this case, divergence of the beam is limited to the effects of diffraction at the beam edges.

Due to the high degree of coherence of a laser beam, it is theoretically possible to focus the beam to the diffraction limit of the wavelength of light. Typically, however, the laser will have a finite beam spread that may be expressed by the simple equations of geometrical optics. As the spot diameter approaches the order of magnitude of the wavelength of light, the spot becomes diffraction limited.

LASER OPTICS IN SURGICAL PRACTICE

Background

Surgeons use lasers on tissues to produce a desirable biological consequence. However, one must realize that when tissues are cut with a laser some real physical problems (Fig 2–9) arise that can interfere with the desirable consequence. It is important to realize what factors can cause these physical problems in order to minimize their effects. However, many of the factors are interrelated. One large problem is the need to reduce the thermal effects to tissues immediately adjacent to the site of laser interaction.

A major factor during laser tissue cutting tissue, while minimizing ther-

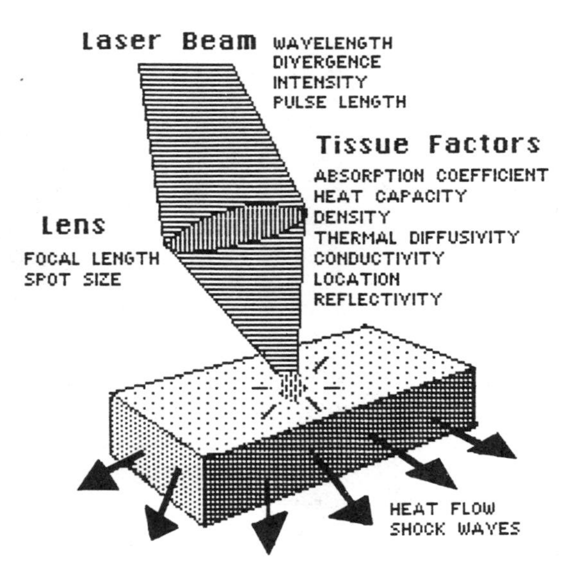

Fig 2–9. Factors relating to laser interactions with tissues. (From Rockwell R.J.: *Laser Safety in Surgery and Medicine.* Cincinnati, Ohio, Rockwell Associates, Inc., 1985. Reproduced by permission.)

mal damage to adjacent tissues, is that the tissue thermal conductivity controls the time required for heat diffusion in tissues. That is, the specific thermal relaxation time of the tissue is involved. This is governed by the equation below that describes the fraction of the absorbed energy (dE) available for heating a given volume:

$$dE = (T_h/T_e)\,(1 - e^{-Te/Th})$$

An inspection of this equation shows that the amount of heat diffusion is limited by the ratios between the duration of the exposure (T_e) and the thermal relaxation time of the tissue (T_h). Since only the first of these, the duration of energy deposition, can be controlled by the surgeon, the importance of using pulsed lasers can be appreciated. The equation also reveals that for a given energy the highest temperatures are reached when the duration is *shorter* than the thermal relaxation time. When $T_e < T_h$ then the exponent of *e,* the base of the natural logarithms, controls the value of dE. By the time the exposure duration is less than one tenth the thermal relaxation time, where $T_h = 10$ μsec (that is, T_e is less than 100 nanoseconds [ns]), essentially all the energy will remain right where it is absorbed long enough to heat just that portion of the material. An even shorter pulse, 10 ns, would allow less than 0.1% of the energy to leave before the peak temperature is reached.

The laser wavelength must be matched as closely as possible to the absorption peak of the material in question to aid in confining the thermal effects to the surface layer. The absorption spectrum of water, as given in Figure 2–10, shows a peak near 2.8 μ, although the absorption is certainly sufficiently high at 10.6 μ to be adequate to make the CO_2 laser work for

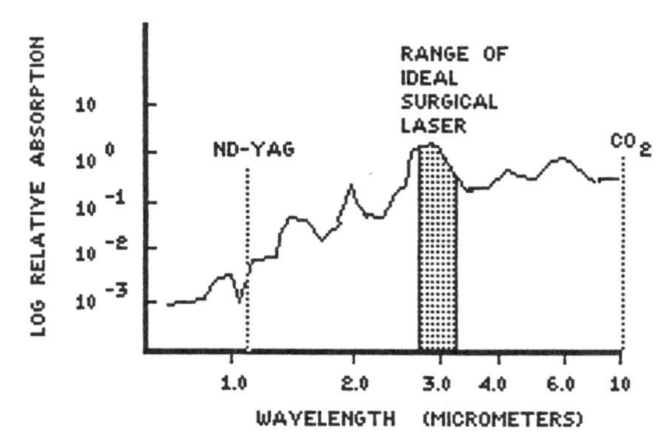

Fig 2–10. Representative absorption spectrum of water. (From Rockwell R.J.: *Laser Safety in Surgery and Medicine.* Cincinnati, Ohio, Rockwell Associates, Inc., 1985. Reproduced by permission.)

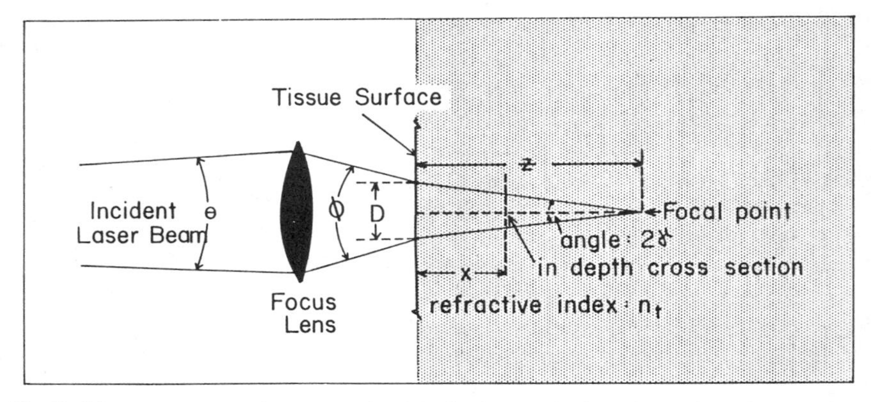

Fig 2–11. Geometrical factors involved in the focus of a laser beam into tissues. (From Rockwell R.J.: *Laser Safety in Surgery and Medicine*. Cincinnati, Ohio, Rockwell Associates, Inc., 1985. Reproduced by permission.)

tissue cutting. However, for the maximum absorption in the shortest tissue distance, a laser in the range from 2.7 to 3.1 μ would also seem to offer some significant advantages.

Physical Concerns

The transverse electromagnetic mode of the laser is an important parameter in determining how the laser beam is focused. The lower the mode pattern, the smaller the spot size at the focal point for a given lens and the longer the depth of focus for the particular spot size. The spot size, or beam diameter, is defined as the point where the beam has fallen to $1/e^2$ of its peak intensity.

Once the surgeon has selected a laser, the only real variable at his or her use is the focal length of the lens placed between the patient and beam. At a given power output, the shorter the focal length, the smaller the spot size, and the greater the irradiance (W/sq cm) of the spot size. A smaller focal length will also decrease the incision width. This last point is very important in surgical applications, since it is the beam focusing that causes the desired biological effect. Knowledge of the exact depth of the laser beam focus is critical in some surgical uses.

As Figure 2–11 shows, a laser beam is also focused by the tissue to a new focal point. The surgeon must allow for the fact that the dense tissue will cause refraction and cause the focus to move deeper in the tissue.

The ability to cut tissues accurately to a specified depth is a very critical factor in laser surgery. A focused beam is held on a given point for sufficient time (t) to ablate the tissue to a desired depth. Once this depth is thought to be achieved, the beam is moved infinitesimally to the next location. If a long focal length lens is used, the variation of focused spot diameter over the cut spot will not be significant, consequently the speed of the cut can be increased—a desirable feature for long operations.

The spot size effected on tissue is almost invariably larger than the optical spot size because of scattering and the thermal conductivity away from the area heated by the focused spot. The effective spot size can be operationally defined as the area of vaporization of resultant heat-affected zone (depending on the application) and the mode of operation of the laser. When used as a cutting tool, the effective spot size is the vaporization zone. When differentially heating the tissue to cause coagulation or tissue shrinkage, the effective spot size is defined as the heat-affected zone.

Surgical Concerns

The term irradiance is very important for laser surgeons since it determines the laser's ability to vaporize, excise, and coagulate tissues of the body. Keep in mind that the desired tissue effects depend on the irradiance (W/sq cm) and *not* simply the laser power (watts) indicated by the laser system power meter.

The optimum irradiance for laser ablation of tissue is often the highest value that can be safely controlled by the surgeons. This concept restricts the damage to healthy tissue in the vicinity of the impact by limiting the beam exposure duration.

The principle may be stated as follows: excess tissue damage is proportional to the time of application of the beam, not to the total power. This principle applies only where the power density is greater than 100 w/sq cm because less than 100 W/sq cm is usually considered ineffectual for surgery. A typical surgical irradiance level might be as high as 5,000 W/sq cm.

Regardless of the laser system used for surgical application, its effects may be broadly categorized as follows:

1. Coagulation
   a. Hemostasis
   b. Necrosis
2. Vaporization
   a. Cutting
   b. Evaporation of tissue.

When used to cut or evaporate tissue, the laser is actually vaporizing cells. The mechanism of vaporization relies on rapid heat transfer from the beam to the cell.

First, the cellular water is heated to at least the boiling point of water. This causes both complete destruction of all cellular proteins and a pressure build-up within the cell (Fig 2–12,A).

The rapid rise in intracellular temperature and pressure causes microexplosion within the cell, throwing off steam vapors and cellular debris (see Fig 2–12,B).

The steam and debris rising from the impact site is seen as the laser plume. This plume remains in the path of the laser beam and the particle fragments flash white hot as they are further heated and carbonized (see Fig 2–12,C.)

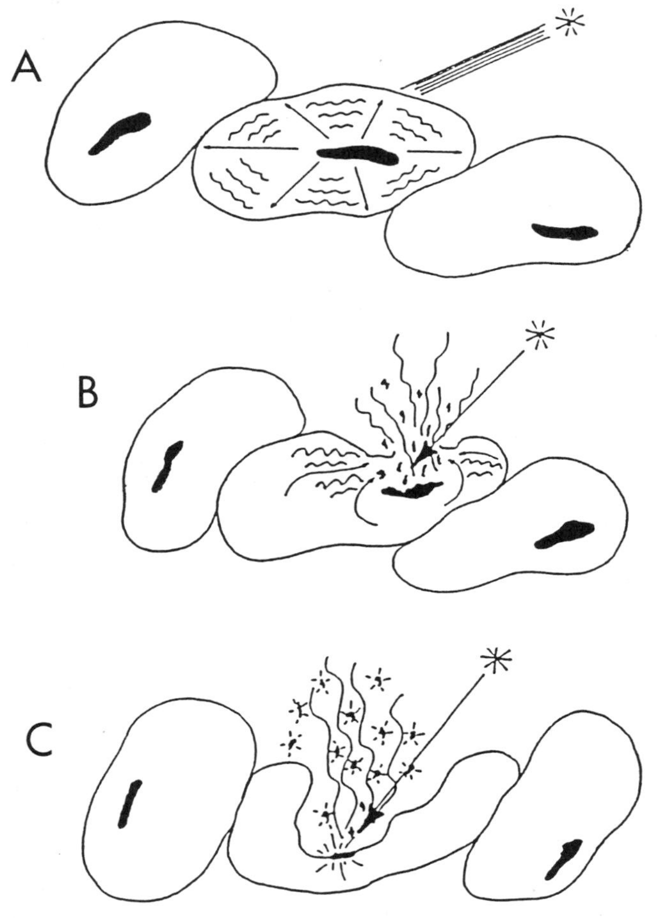

Fig 2–12. Laser-tissue interaction: **(A)** beam onto tissue, **(B)** tissue alteration, **(C)** origin of the laser plume gasses. (From Rockwell R.J.: *Laser Safety in Surgery and Medicine.* Cincinnati, Ohio, Rockwell Associates, Inc., 1985. Reproduced by permission.)

With a CO_2 laser, for example, the zone of damage produced is very limited, both laterally and in depth. A CO_2 laser beam, for example, is completely absorbed within about 0.1 mm depth in water. The lateral zone of damage extends less than 0.5 mm and is composed of three distinct zones around the incision or crater: (1) the inner carbonized zone; (2) the middle dessicated zone; and (3) the outer edematous zone.

Because of the precise localization of the CO_2 laser beam effects, as well as the sealing effects of the beam, surrounding tissue exhibits minimal edema, scarring, or stenosis.

Whether used with a handpiece or microscope, the focused beam is swept across the incision line. The depth of cut depends on both irradiance and time.

By moving the focusing lens away slightly, the incident beam irradiance is quickly reduced (due to the larger spot size) and one will minimize the tissue effects to produce tissue evaporation or coagulation (when at lower power or larger spots).

When used with a microscope, the manipulation is slightly different. The working distance from the tissue is now set by the objective lens of the microscope. Adjusting the spot size of the laser beam now involves changing lenses by a rotating thumbwheel. The beam is manually directed by a micromanipulator.

To use the laser-microscope to cut or vaporize small areas, the spot needs to be at its smallest size, and have highest irradiance. This is accomplished by matching the laser lens to the microscope objective lens: i.e., a 300-mm objective, a 300-mm laser lens; a 400-mm objective, a 400 mm-laser lens, etc. When changing the laser lens, one needn't keep looking at the thumbwheel labels, as the difference in size of the spot can easily be seen through the microscope.

"Prefocus" refers to the condition of focusing the microscope into this tissue. In this case, the laser spot on the surface of the tissue will be larger than when it is in focus and can be used for debulking tissue and, at lower powers, coagulating. Since the laser focus is *behind* the tissue surface, one needs to be acutely aware of structures behind the impact point. If the laser were fixed in the continuous mode over the same spot, it would burn faster as it penetrated because of the underlying focal point. Also, if one is positioned over a delicate structure such as an artery, it is possible to pierce a hole when using the prefocus selection. Ordinarily though, except for higher powers and/or very proximate structures, the prefocused position is satisfactory for evaporating tissue and coagulating.

The prefocus position will not effect underlying tissue with the CO_2 laser until everything in front is vaporized. This is not true of a Nd:YAG laser, which can effect underlying tissues that are not in the surgeon's view.

A partially defocused position can be used in much the same way as the prefocus except that the focal point of the laser is now *in front of* the tissue. This means that if the laser were fixed in the continuous mode over the same spot, it would burn slower as it penetrated because the spot is spreading. When used in the pulsed mode, it may be impossible to distinguish between the defocused and the prefocus condition.

When no lens is used, the beam maintains the same diameter as the incident beam. This causes a spot that is excellent for coagulating and, at higher powers, for rapidly evaporating broad areas of tissue.

Time is also a very useful tool for manipulating the tissue effects of the beam. One can pulse the beam rather than using the continuous mode. Even though the foot pedal can be pumped when the laser is in continuous, the amount of control this gives is negligible compared with an electronically pulsed mode. The effect of decreasing pulse times is equivalent to decreasing power settings. The biological effect of 10 W at a 0.2-s pulse will be roughly equivalent to 20 W at 0.1 s.*

The unit of the joule describes the total energy dose of the beam delivered into the tissue and is the product of the power and time.

Consequently, manipulating the pulse duration is equivalent to changing energy. Lasers that are used exclusively or primarily in the pulsed mode such as ruby or Nd:YAG will have pulse outputs expressed in joules.

Another way to manipulate the time of the impact through the microscope is to quickly move or wiggle the spot back and forth over the tissue. The faster it moves, the less the effect on the tissue. A focused spot used at lower powers can be used to make a slow incision. If this same focused spot is then moved quickly, it can be used to evaporate tissue. Moved even more quickly, the spot is used to coagulate and achieve hemostasis in an area of small bleeders. In this way one can obtain several different effects without having to rotate to a different lens. When evaporating large areas or coagulating an entire field, the spot needs to be quickly moved back and forth in a crisscross pattern.

The laser is generally used to do one of the following three procedures: cut, evaporate, coagulate.

Cutting Concepts

When used for cutting, the beam is used with the spot in focus on the tissue (smallest spot size). Preciseness of the laser beam and localization of damage are two advantages of this condition. The thermal effects of the beam to seal vessels and lymphatics as it cuts creates a dry surgical field that makes many procedures easier and quicker.

The depth of cut is determined by irradiance and exposure time. The

*This actually depends on irradiance and time, not simply power and time.

higher the irradiance applied and the slower the speed the spot is moved across an incision, the deeper it will cut (Fig 2–13).

Practice is the only way to learn the "feel" of cutting accurately and safely with the focused laser beam. Especially distracting in the surgeon's initial laser experience is the lack of tactile feedback to gauge the depth of cut. Experience will allow eventually for increased power requirements and methods for protecting adjacent tissue will lead to more speed and precision.

Incisions with the laser heal much the same way as a surgical scalpel incision. Histologically, the scars are identical at 20 to 30 days even though the healing mechanism is slightly delayed. Laser incisions may undergo more rapid re-epithelialization, but its tensile strength is less than scalpel until 30 to 40 days when they are identical. In practice many surgeons say they see no clinical difference between the two wounds.

Evaporation Concepts

The evaporation of tissue can be performed with a prefocused, partially defocused, or totally defocused spot. Small areas may be evaporated with a focused spot, but large areas tend to get ridges and rows in them if evaporated in this manner. Evaporation is an advantage in debulking tumors or precisely removing tissue (tumor) one cell layer at a time from delicate structures such as nerves or vessels. Ablative lesions may also be placed with a defocused or unfocused beam.

Coagulation Concepts

Even though the beam coagulates vessels up to 0.5 mm instantaneously as it cuts, it is necessary to defocus the spot to coagulate larger vessels up to 2

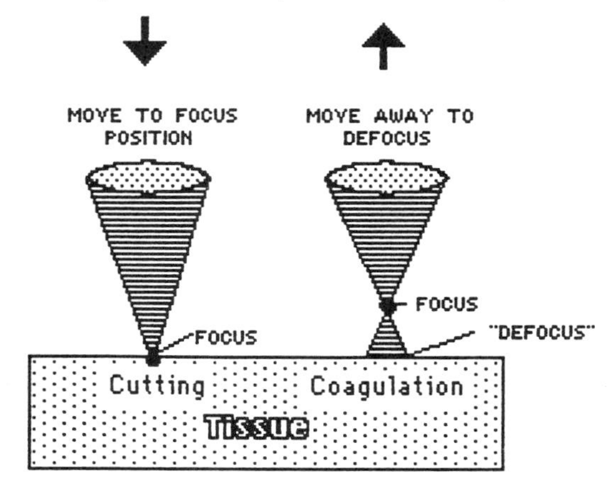

Fig 2–13. Beam focus variations in laser cutting and coagulation techniques. (From Rockwell R.J.: *Laser Safety in Surgery and Medicine*. Cincinnati, Ohio, Rockwell Associates, Inc., 1985. Reproduced by permission.)

mm. When using a micromanipulator, this same effect can be achieved by very quickly moving the spot back and forth over a vessel. A combination of low powers, large spots, and pulsed exposures will best accomplish this goal. Laser evaporation may continue in a bloody field by use of constant suction. One must lase directly on the vessel and tissue that is not covered by blood. Lasering through blood only makes a black, sticky coagulum with continued bleeding underneath. The use of a nonreflective suction tubing for removal of blood and smoke can facilitate continuous removal of tumor and other tissues.

Larger veins, 2 to 5 mm in diameter, may be coagulated with the laser by moving a defocused beam slowly over the vessel. The effect is to shrink the vessel so much that its lumen is obliterated. The beam may then focus and the vessel can be cut.

The CO_2 surgical laser is best employed as a vaporizing function rather than for coagulation. It does have some very beneficial coagulative properties such as sealing capillaries and shrinking up larger veins, but it is not intended to function as an in-depth tissue coagulator. A Nd:YAG laser is, perhaps, better suited for in-depth coagulation due to the lower absorption in tissues at the 1.06-μm laser wavelength. Refinement of the Nd:YAG and CO_2 laser may provide the necessary precision to weld arteries for microsurgery of malformations and anastomosis of small vessels.

Irradiance and Beam Cross Section

Since the beam irradiance is so important in laser surgery, let us examine this concept further. Obviously, irradiance is a function of spot size and applied power. Spot size, from previous discussions, is determined by the focal length of the lens, laser mode, and the laser wavelength. Thus, to have a small spot size one needs a short focal length lens, short laser wavelengths (i.e., argon rather than CO_2), and laser modes that produce relatively even energy distribution over the beam area. Figure 2–7 shows a plot of the intensity produced by a so-called TEM_{oo} laser compared with the first order (donut) mode. When the power level is not distributed in the TEM_{oo} manner, it is said to be in a higher mode distribution. The surgical importance of this type of distribution would be analogous to cutting with a dull knife.

The practical use of such information becomes clear when comparing surgical cutting or coagulation techniques (see Fig 2–13). Because the two techniques are so different, the beam must be manipulated by adjusting the power setting *and* spot size. When this is done, the following becomes apparent.

The cutting process demands rapid energy absorption in tissue. However, to prevent potential damage to adjacent tissues, the laser can be emitted in short bursts.

When a laser beam is focused by a lens on a tissue for a given time, the overall zone of the thermal defect created by the beam is determined by the thermal processes that occur during *and following* the time the laser is actually on the site. There is a minimum temperature required to create certain effects. At lower irradiance levels, the minimal requirement will be produced only by the central part of the focal spot. As the output is increased, the percentage of the Gaussian beam distribution containing this minimum irradiance becomes larger and the diameter of the tissue effects will increase. Hence the "spot size" dimension is very important in the eventual laser-tissue interaction.

USE OF FIBEROPTICS

Background

Fiberoptics applications began in 19th century England when John Tyndall discovered that light was guided along an arc in a moving stream of water. From that crude beginning the field has grown into a multimillion dollar industry with applications in most scientific fields including medicine. Since fiberoptics are now used in numerous medical laser units, it is helpful for surgeons to have a basic familiarization with fiberoptics.

The term *fiberoptics* is the name given to a small diameter glass or plastic waveguide that transmits optical radiation. Normally, this waveguide is in the shape of a round elongated rod. Fiberoptics transmit optical energy from the entrance to the exit with minimal loss of signal.

Optical fibers transmit light by causing the rays to undergo multiple internal reflections inside the fiber. Ideally, one wants a fiberoptic bundle to accept all the light incident on its end surface and to transmit this light perfectly to the other end. Historically, intensity losses do occur in the fiber if it were quite large. However, the major advance in fiberoptics technology has been maximizing the amount of light transmitted by using fibers having extremely low losses.

Intensity losses of various kinds occur both at the end surfaces and along the length of the fiber. For example, only certain rays (those incident on the end of the fiber within a certain range of angles) can be transmitted through a fiber of any appreciable length. Other rays will be lost, and hence some of the incident intensity. The range of angles at which the fiber can accept light can vary widely depending on the materials of which the fiber core and cladding are made. A quantity called "numerical aperture" is used to describe this range and is thus an indirect measure of the ability of the fiber to transmit light.

Another part of the incident light is lost by being reflected off the end surfaces. This "Fresnel reflection" accounts for the loss of from 1% to 9% of the light that the numerical aperture indicates the fiber should accept.

In addition to end losses, they also have line losses (i.e., losses along the length of the fiber). Line losses are caused by absorption of some of the light by the core material and by imperfect internal reflections. Line losses depend strongly on the length of the fiber.

Laser surgeons are currently using fibers to transmit visible and near infrared radiation. Such fibers are about 200 to 600 μm in diameter, and are lightweight, flexible, and rugged. These fibers are excellent for viewing and treating internal procedures through endoscopes.

While good fiberoptics exist in the medical field for use with various lasers, there are at present no commercially available fibers for use with CO_2 lasers. Therefore, surgical CO_2 lasers are equipped with articulated arms. An articulated arm utilizes a set of mirrors repeatedly reflect the beam by 90°. The mirrors are held together by means of hollow metallic tubes, about 0.5 in. in diameter, through which the beam propagates, and the entire configuration can be pointed almost arbitrarily due to the freedom provided by rotating joints that incorporate the mirrors.

The laser propagating through this arrangement is typically 6 mm in diameter, and, if the arm is properly aligned, the beam does not interact at all with the walls. The tubes have only a mechanical support role, and do not act as waveguides. The beam going out of such an articulated arm is virtually the same as the laser output beam. This feature plus their high-power handling capability is a major advantage of articulated arms. On the negative side, the large diameter and stiffness of each link render articulated arms awkward to move. Furthermore, the relatively large number of components necessary to make versatile arms means that alignment is critical and the arms can be out of alignment with some frequency.

TYPES OF SURGICAL LASERS

Introduction

In general, there are three major laser types used in surgical applications: argon, CO_2, and Nd:YAG. They can all operate in several different ways. The lasers are known by the material used for the lasing medium and are designated by the emitted wavelength and output power. The output may be delivered in a single pulse, in a series of pulses, or as a continuous level of power as determined in Table 2–1.

Two parameters, wavelength and the power-time (energy) characteristics, are important to the proper laser selection. The wavelength of the laser and the spectral absorption of the tissue at the laser wavelength determines

TABLE 2–1.—SURGICAL LASER SYSTEMS AVAILABLE

TYPE	MODE OF OPERATION	OUTPUT (WATTS)	REPETITION RATE (HERTZ)	PULSE WIDTH (MSEC)
CO_2	Continuous	0.1–150	. . .	. . .
10.6 μ	Pulsed	25 watts (avg.)	1–300	$0.1–250 \times 10^{-3}$
Argon	Continuous	0.01–20	. . .	. . .
0.488 μ	Pulsed	0.01–20 (avg.)	1–250	$0.1–500 \times 10^{-3}$
Nd-Yag	Continuous	0.5–100	. . .	. . .
1.06 μ	Q-switched	500 (peak)	1,000–5,0000	$150–300 \times 10^{-9}$

the percentage of the beam *absorbed* by the tissue. The higher the absorption, the smaller the penetration depth (Fig 2–14).

Figure 2–14 contrasts the absorption effects of different lasers in three important biological materials. Note that tissues containing melanin and hemoglobin absorb argon wavelengths very strongly, but that higher levels of irradiance are required from argon lasers to vaporize or coagulate unpigmented tissue. On the other hand, Nd:YAG laser wavelengths are neither appreciably absorbed or scattered in tissues. As a result, higher power Nd:YAG levels are needed to produce tissue coagulation. Since the Nd:YAG

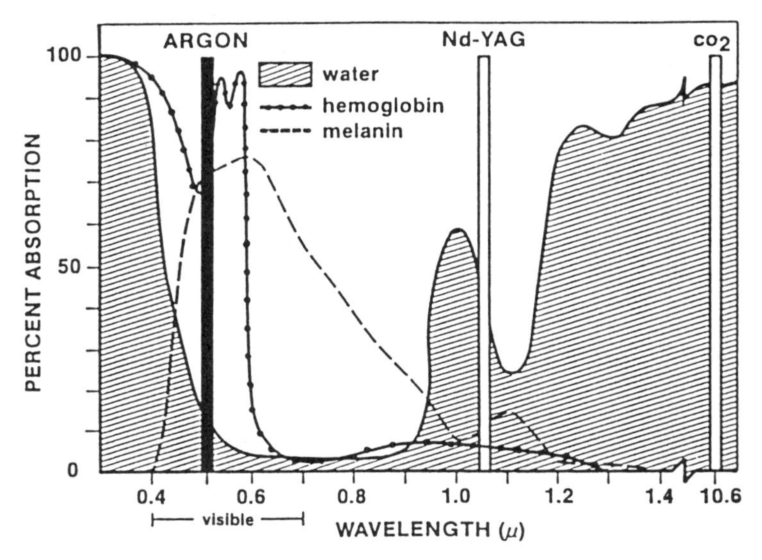

Fig 2–14. Absorption spectra in hemoglobin, melanin and water. Note variations at wavelengths of Argon (0.488–0.514 μm), Nd-YAG (1.064 μm) and the CO_2 (10.6 μm) lasers. (From Rockwell R.J.: *Laser Safety in Surgery and Medicine*. Cincinnati, Ohio, Rockwell Associates, Inc., 1985. Reproduced by permission.)

TABLE 2–2.—TYPICAL PENETRATION DEPTH OF MEDICAL LASERS

LASER	WAVELENGTH (NM)	DEPTH (MM)
Argon	488–514	0.84
Nd-Yag	1,060	4.2
CO_2	10,600	0.23

laser is not absorbed as well, it has a higher penetration depth. Finally, the CO_2 wavelengths are shown to be entirely absorbed in a few hundred micron thickness of the water in soft tissue. As a result, CO_2 laser radiation is excellent in surgical procedure, since absorption is independent on tissue color and little heat conduction arises due to absorption in water.

Table 2–2 shows the penetration depth associated with all the major medical lasers. The penetration depth is that tissue depth necessary to absorb 99% of the incident radiation and is of prime interest in choosing a particular laser for a given procedure.

The power-time characteristics are important for determining the amount of tissue vaporization or coagulation. An unfocused laser beam typically does not provide sufficient irradiance to cause the temperature rise desired for most surgical (cutting) applications. The beam diameter of an unfocused laser typically ranges from a few millimeters to 2 cm and is suited for some dermatological applications where a broad beam may be desired.

Most users, however, require focusing the output of the laser. Focusing the laser of a given power increases the watts per unit area delivered to the tissue, thereby increasing the effect on the tissue.

In a pulsed laser, the power-time characteristics are all important, and typically, the output specifications are expressed in terms of the pulse energy (joules). When the output beam is continuously pulsed, the important specification is usually expressed in terms of average power (watts), pulse repetition rate (pps) and single pulse duration (seconds). In addition, the peak power (watts) of the individual pulse is also often specified.

CO_2

From the standpoint of medical applications, the CO_2 laser offers both high power and high efficiency at a far infrared wavelength. The CO_2 laser is the important example of a class of lasers referred to as molecular lasers. Molecules have a more complicated structure with corresponding energy levels that relate to oscillating or vibrating motions of the entire molecular structure. The atoms in the molecule can vibrate relative to each other, and the entire molecule can rotate.

The energy level structure of a molecule, such as CO_2 is far more complex than that of an atom (ion) because there are more "energy-exchange" mechanisms. In molecules, there are three such mechanisms, corresponding to electronic, vibrational, and rotational motion.

From the safety viewpoint, the CO_2 radiation does not penetrate the ocular media of the eye and is far less of an ocular hazard at the same power level than either an Argon or Nd:YAG laser. It should be noted that one aims the CO_2 laser using a low-power He-Ne laser (which is red visible light). Sometimes there is a problem seeing the red light on certain tissues. Hence, the He-Ne should be capable of varying intensity and beam size. In some cases one might pulse its output for ease of observation.

Argon

Argon ion lasers produce the highest visible power levels and have up to ten lasing wavelengths in the blue-green portion of the spectra. These lasers are normally rated by the power level produced by the six wavelengths, from 514.5 to 457.9 nm. The most prominent argon wavelengths are the 514.5 and 488.0 nm-lines. The wavelengths outside the visible range are only available by changing mirrors.

The rare gases, helium, neon, argon, xenon, and krypton, have completed electronic shells and, consequently, do not normally combine chemically with other elements. Although their chemical usefulness is limited, they have exhibited remarkable ability to attain stimulated emission.

However, with the exception of neon, none of the neutral rare gases are very useful as practical high average power lasers. The other noble gases, when used as laser media, must be ionized by electron collisions. The resulting ion is excited by further electron collisions and an inverted population of the ion energy levels is achieved. To ionize the noble gas atoms, a large amount of current (on the order of 15 to 40 amps) must be passed through the discharge tube.

The high current through the small bore of an argon ion laser demands refractory materials that can withstand the intense heating caused by the highly excited gas. The high current causes a pumping of the argon ions toward the cathode and the electrons toward the anode. Because the mobility of the ions is much less than the mobility of the electrons, the ions pile up at the cathode. There they are neutralized and then diffuse slowly into the bore again. If nothing is done to counteract this slow diffusion, the discharge ceases.

To dissipate the large amount of generated heat, argon ion laser tubes are water cooled. Although some lasers have separate heat exchanges, most use tap water. This results in some of the greatest operating problems, for if the water is not flowing with sufficient rate, boiling occurs along the tube. The popping and fizzing causes cavity vibrations and these in turn cause amplitude and frequency instabilities.

Simple, pulsed versions of argon ion lasers also are available. Because the duty cycle ("on" time divided by the time between pulses) is low, the heat energy generated is small, and usually only convective cooling is needed. The average power output may be as high as several watts, although the peak powers can be as high as several kilowatts. Pulse widths are approximately 5 to 50 μsec, with repetition rates as high as 60 Hz.

Nd:YAG

Nd:YAG lasers belong to the class of solid state lasers. Solid state lasers occupy a unique place in laser development. The first operational laser medium was a crystal of pink ruby; since that time, the term *solid state laser* usually has been used to describe a laser whose active medium is a crystal doped with an impurity ion. Solid state lasers are rugged, simple to maintain, and capable of generating high powers.

In all cases, the active medium of a solid state laser consists of an insulator crystal and a dopant impurity. The insulatory crystal atoms do not participate directly in the lasing action, but serve as a host lattice in which the dopant resides. The dopant is an impurity added deliberately to the crystal lattice at the time of growth. Most of the dopants are the heavy multielectron atoms, which have strong absorption bands in the visible spectrum. When the dopant is free to move in a gaseous discharge, rather than constrained in the lattice, the lowest energy levels all have the same energy and are said to be degenerate.

Although solid state lasers offer some unique advantages over gas lasers, crystals are not ideal cavities or perfect laser media. Real crystals contain refractive index variations that distort the wavefront and mode structure of the laser. High-power operation causes thermal expansion of the crystal that alters the effective cavity dimensions and thus changes the modes. The laser crystals are cooled by forced air or liquids, particularly for high repetition rates.

The most striking aspect of solid state lasers is that the output is usually not continuous, but consists of a large number of often separated power bursts. Because of this spiked output, the coherence length of solid-state lasers is frequently only several centimeters, quite poor compared with gas lasers. Although this poor coherence length makes solid-state lasers unsuitable for many applications, they are unsurpassed for producing intense bursts of visible light from a relatively small laser.

COMMENTS

The preceding review of laser systems emphasized a few of the "most common" laser types used in surgery that are generally available commercially. These lasers are by no means representative of the vast number of different lasers that are manufactured. This brief overview should reveal that even these most common laser types produce a wide range of output levels and specific beam characteristics that are dependent in a complex way on the particular laser media and the manner in which it is operated. This makes a general broad comparison of all laser devices a difficult, if not impossible, task.

The broad spectrum of different lasers does impose serious problems in providing safety protection for users, since the advantages introduced by such a broad spectrum is, of itself, a disadvantage when attempting to provide a uniform "all-purpose" laser safety code. As a result, the personnel using lasers, whether in the laboratory or in a medical environment, as well as the health officers responsible for enforcement of a laser safety regulations, will require more detailed and specific data regarding the following: (1) the operational parameters of the laser(s) in use; (2) the safe exposure criteria for each laser; and (3) the correct protective devices necessary for these lasers.

Similarly, those responsible for establishing levels for safe exposures as well as those who manufacture protection devices must also keep pace with the advances in the technology.

RADIATION CONCERNS OF SURGICAL LASERS

General Overview

Laser radiation of sufficient intensity and exposure time can cause irreversible damage to the skin and eye of humans. The principal cause of tissue damage is thermal in nature. The process is one where the tissue proteins are denatured due to the temperature rise in tissues following absorption of laser energy. The thermal damage process is generally associated with lasers operating at exposure times greater than 10 μsec and in the wavelength region from the near ultraviolet to the far infrared ($0.315 - 10^3$ μm).

Other damage mechanisms have also been demonstrated for other specific wavelength ranges and/or exposure times. For example, photochemical reactions are the principal cause of tissue damage following exposures to either actinic ultraviolet radiation (0.200 − 0.315 μm) for any exposure time or "short-wave" visible radiation (0.4 − 0.55 μm) when exposures are greater than 10 seconds. Tissue damage may also be caused by thermally induced acoustic-shock waves following exposures to very short-time laser exposures (submicrosecond).

The principle tissue damage mechanism for repetitively pulsed or scanned laser exposures is still in some question. Current evidence would indicate that the major mechanism is a thermal process wherein the effects of the individual pulses are additive. There seems to be a different damage process for repetitively pulsed laser exposures when the individual pulses are shorter than 10 μsec than occurs when the pulses are greater than 10 μsec in duration.

Skin and Internal Organs

The laser skin surface makes this structure readily accessible to both acute and chronic exposures to all forms of optical radiation that can produce skin damage of varying degrees. Numerous different types of lasers have been explored rather extensively for the therapy of skin disorders in humans. Certainly, skin injury is of lesser importance than eye damage, however, with the expanding use of higher-power laser systems, the unprotected skin of personnel using lasers may be exposed more frequently to hazardous levels. Table 2–3 shows the 50% maximum skin reaction level for several laser types.

The structural inhomogenities of the skin can cause internal scattering of optical radiation in tissues. As a result, there will be multiple internal reflections in addition to absorption and transmission of the incident laser beam. For the most common laser sources in the 0.3 to 1.0-μm range, almost 99% of the radiation penetrating the skin will be absorbed in at least the outer 4 mm of tissue.

For wavelengths greater than 0.4 μm, the reaction of the skin to absorbed optical radiation is essentially that of a thermal coagulation necrosis. This type of injury can be produced by any optical radiation source of similar parameters and is, therefore, not a reaction specific to laser radiation. It is similar in causality and clinical appearance to the tissues reaction of the deep electrical burn. For pulsed laser irradiation, including exposures of the picosecond domain, there may be other secondary reactions in the tissues. Studies have shown that the volume of vaporized tissues produced by high-level irradiation with laser pulses in the msec domain can backscatter a significant portion of the incident energy. This effectively reduces the amount of absorbed radiation in the tissues.

The principal thermal effects of laser exposure depend on the following factors:

1. Absorption and scattering coefficients of the tissues at the laser wavelength.

TABLE 2–3.—MINIMAL REACTIVE DOSE LEVELS FOR SKIN

LASER TYPE	RADIANT EXPOSURE* (J/k²)	EXPOSURE TIME (SECONDS)
Ruby (unpigmented skin)	11–20	2.5×10^{-3}
@ 0.694 μ (pigmented skin)	2.2–6.9	
Ruby: Q-switched @ 0.694 μ	0.25–0.24	75×10^{-9}
Argon ion gas (cw) @ 0.514 μ	4.0–8.2	1.0
Carbon dioxide (cw) @ 10.6 μ	2.8	1.0
Nd glass (long pulse) @ 1.06 μ	2.5–5.7	75×10^{-9}
Nd-YAG: Q-switched @ 1.064 μ	46–78	1.0
Excimer (xenon chloride) @ 0.308 μ	0.5	—

*Evaluated at 50% probability levels for minimal tissue reaction except for excimer which is the minimal level for tissue ablation.

2. Irradiance or radiant exposure of the laser beam.

3. Duration of the exposure and pulse repetition characteristics, if applicable.

4. Extent of the local vascular flow.

5. Size of the area irradiated.

The results of studies on the exposure levels required to produce minimal reactions in the human skin for six common laser types emitting in the visible and infrared is summarized in Figure 2–15. The variations, or spread, in the data were found to be directly related to the degree of absorption.

The Eye

The principal hazard associated with laser radiation is exposure to the eye. This is particularly important in the visible and near-infrared spectral regions (0.400–1.400 μm). There are, however, other serious potential hazards in other spectral regions, as outlined in the following sections.

The eye may be conceptually considered as a slightly flattened globe that is transparent to the light passing through an aperture (pupil) and that has an efficient light absorber on the inside (retinal surface), opposite the

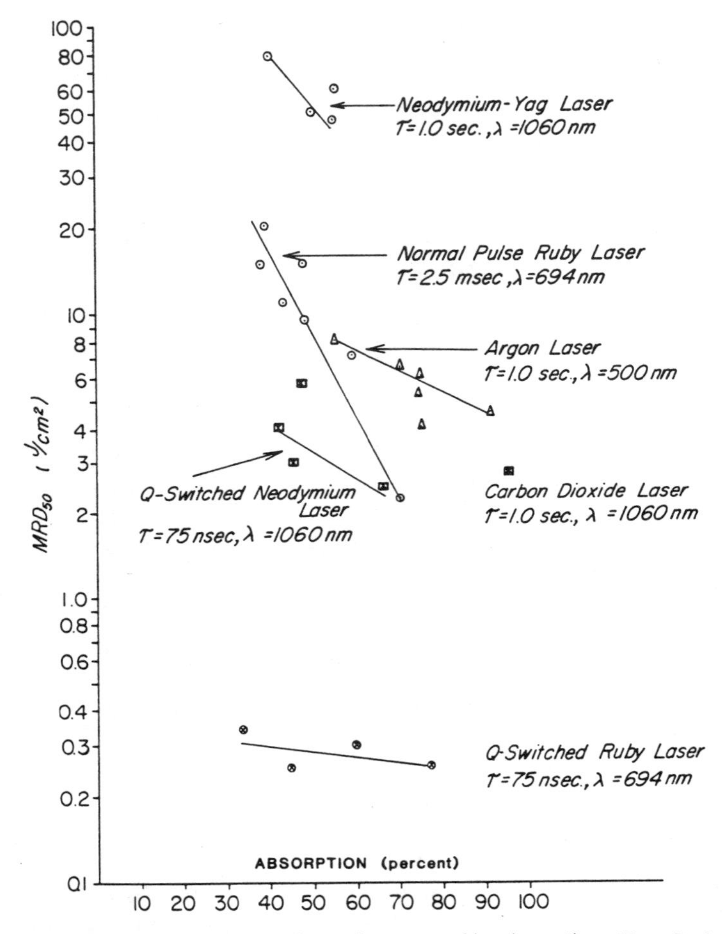

Fig 2–15. Minimal reactive dose dependence on skin absorption. (From Rockwell R.J.: *Laser Safety in Surgery and Medicine*. Cincinnati, Ohio, Rockwell Associates, Inc., 1985. Reproduced by permission.)

aperture. The transparent region of the eye includes several structures that operate to control the exposure to the retina.

The cornea, the transparent window, is the primary refracting structure of the eye. Because of the differences in refractive indices of air and the cornea, more than 80% of the refraction of light takes place as the light enters the eye. Between the cornea and the lens is one of the two chambers of the eye. The aqueous chamber contains the aqueous fluid.

The lens is the dynamic refractive medium in the eye, and is responsible for the range of focus of the eye. The retina is the light-absorbing structure of the eye, containing the neural receptors that initiate the vision process. A blind spot in the retinal surface is located at the point where the optic nerve enters into the eye. The fovea is the portion of the retina that is most sensitive to detail and that discriminates color. This structure fills an angle of approximately 2° in the central portion of the retina. The fovea is located in a small dip in the center of the area called the macula lutea. The macula fills an area of about 1 mm diameter.

The various structures of the eye transmit, reflect, and absorb optical energy. The effects of laser exposure on the retina are influenced by the transmission losses of the ocular media. Figure 2–16 shows the transmittance of the ocular media. It is apparent from this figure that retinal effects can be anticipated only for laser wavelengths between 0.400 μm and 1.4 μm. Outside that range, structures other than the retina are affected. The retinal effects of visible optical radiation are also influenced by the size of the retinal image and the time duration of the laser exposure.

Early in the history of lasers, it was recognized that lasers had great potential for causing retinal injury. The reason was that a laser could produce retinal intensities that were orders of magnitude greater than conventional light sources, and, in fact, brighter than the sun.

The optical system of the eye, like any optical system, will have a limi-

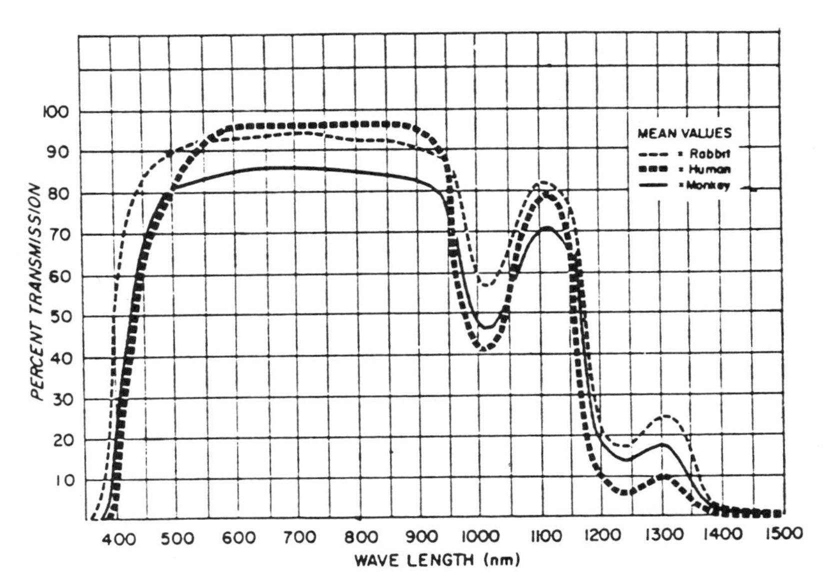

Fig 2–16. Transmittance of ocular media. (From Rockwell R.J.: *Laser Safety in Surgery and Medicine*. Cincinnati, Ohio, Rockwell Associates, Inc., 1985. Reproduced by permission.)

tation (called the diffraction limit) on the smallest size of image it may resolve and focus. To determine the effect of a source imaged on the retina, it is necessary to know the retinal image size. A large amount of the research on retinal burns indicates that the size of the source is an important variable. For a first approximation, one can show that a laser with a 1-m rad beam spread will produce a retinal spot of approximate size of 17 μm.

If an unaccommodated eye (an eye focused at infinity) views a collimated source such as a distant star in the night sky or a laser, a "point" image *should* be produced on the retina. In practice, however, a true point image of that light source is *not* produced. The optical system of the eye, or any optical instrument, has certain limitations caused by diffraction that will cause the light rays passing through an aperture to bend. The aperture of an optical system is the edge that produces the diffraction. The aperture in the eye is the iris. If a laser beam is larger than the pupil, diffraction of the beam occurs at the edge of the iris.

If the beam is smaller than the pupil, spherical aberrations and forward scattering cause the "point" image to spread. In general, the larger the pupil, the smaller the point spread and the greater the magnification factor or concentration of light at the retina as compared with the irradiance at the cornea. Estimations of the magnification factor, based on diffraction effects only, range from 10^5 to 10^7 for pupil diameters between 2 and 7 mm.

The location of the exposure in the eye determines the degree of incapacitation from a retinal injury. The fovea (the central 2° of the visual field) is the region of the retina that is most sensitive to visual detail. The remainder of the retina, the parafovea to the peripheral retina, is increasingly less sensitive to light.

The parafovea and peripheral retina, however, are not as sensitive and do not contribute significantly to fine detail in the vision process. Therefore, any injury to the fovea will severely reduce visual function as regards to visual detail and resolution. An injury to the parafovea or peripheral retina is less incapacitating and may be undetectable from a functional point of view.

When viewing an extended source, such as the reflection of a laser from a diffuse highly reflective surface, the geometry of the situation results in a retinal image that is of constant brightness (constant retinal irradiance) until the observer moves away so far that the eye can no longer resolve the spot of the laser light. At this point a critical image size is reached. When this occurs, the brightness will stay constant or decrease in value. Retinal spot size effects are related to the differential effects of conduction of heat away from the image, which are a function of both exposure time and image size. For long exposures, the large and small image size damage thresholds are different because of thermal conduction.

LASER SAFETY REGULATIONS AND PRACTICES—THE ANSI Z136 STANDARDS

Control measures can be employed to reduce ocular and skin exposure to hazardous laser levels as well as other hazards associated with the operation of laser devices. There are four basic categories of control measures useful in laser environments. These categories are engineering controls, personal protective equipment, administrative procedural controls, and special controls (Table 2–4).

Several recent incidences during laser surgery procedures may suggest a need for more comprehensive understanding of the existing recommended safety procedures and, in addition, training of the laser surgery personnel. New detailed recommendations for laser safety have been published by the American National Standards Institute (ANSI) in the publication *For the Safe Use of Lasers* ANSI Z136.1 on which existing federal and the new proposed model state legislation are based.

TABLE 2–4.—Basic Laser Controls for Safe Laser Use

Engineering Controls	*Administrative and Procedural Controls*
Protective housing	Laser safety officer
Interlocks-housing	Written work practices (SOPs)
Beam enclosures	Output limitations
Beam shutter or attenuator	Education and training
Remote interlock connector	Maintenance
Key switch control	Alignment procedures
Viewing optics and windows	Personal protective devices
Service panels	Spectator limitations
Emission delay	Warning signs (caution/danger)
Warning system	
Controlled Areas	
Indoor	
Temporary	
Outdoor	
Remote firing and monitoring	
Equipment labels	
Personal Protective Equipment	*Special Controls*
Eyewear	IR and UV requirements (nonvisible beams)
Factors	Demonstrations involving the general public (laser-light shows)
Optical density	Fiberoptic systems
Transmission	Responsibility of manufacturers
Identification	Repair and maintenance
Fit and comfort	Modification of laser systems
Clothing	
Other	

The American National Standards Institute (ANSI) is an organization in which expert volunteers participate in committees to determine industry consensus standards in various fields. Laser safety regulations are based on this standard. In addition, the ANSI Z136 exposure criteria standard served as the basis for the Laser Safety chapter of the WHO and for the TC-76 Standard on Lasers of the International Electrotechnical Commission (IEC). It has, therefore, an international scope. The standard is more devised for the *user* than for the manufacturers of lasers, although many manufacturers also adhere to the standard during production.

Under development at this time is a separate edition of the ANSI Z136 standard that pertains only to appropriate controls for medical lasers. This edition, denoted as "Laser Safety in the Health Care Environment" (Z136.3) will address concerns associated with training, necessary equipment safety features, eye protection requirements, confirmation of power monitor measurements, programmed equipment audit, and appropriate area controls. Since most surgical lasers are Class IV systems, one can also expect Z136.3 to cover with control measures necessary for the surgical OR. This edition should be ready for publication by the end of 1986. Until its publication, this safety information will focus on existing Z136 requirements that are pertinent to the medical laser area.

Great responsibility has been delegated to the management in regard to laser safety and training programs. For surgical lasers installed in a hospital, the administration has this management responsibility. For office surgical users, it is the physician/owner.

To appreciate details of the ANSI Z136 standard and how it would apply to the surgical institutions, the following sections from the standard will convey its meaning. (Note that some sections are not in the same continuity as the standard.)

CONTROL MEASURES AS SPECIFIED IN ANSI Z136.1

The ANSI Z136.1 laser safety standard applies to the wide field of laser technology and is not specifically devised for laser surgery. Some of the regulations, such as the recommended door interlocks, are difficult to employ in the OR. The traffic in and out of the OR, especially during major surgical procedures, is frequent, and an interlock system could conceivably interfere with the surgical procedure. Under the 1980 language of the standard, "unexpected entry" into a surgical OR would not frequently occur during a surgical procedure, since entry by nurses and ancillary OR staff is expected and anticipated during the procedure. Under these conditions, then, strict adherence is required to the requirements for training and personal protective equipment for all personnel entering the OR as well as for all personnel in the OR. The revised 1986 version of the standard will also recommend barriers be used in the OR door pathway if hazardous levels of laser radiation could escape upon door opening.

In regard to medical surveillance, examination of the cornea alone is probably sufficient for the CO_2 lasers used in the OR. The CO_2 laser, operating at the far infrared wavelength of 10.6 μm does not usually present a retinal hazard to the user. Protective clothing is an important consideration in the OR. The surgical field should be draped with moist gauze or towel. Paper drapes and gowns ignite readily and should be avoided.

The required control measures necessary for medical lasers as detailed in the ANSI-Z136.1 1980 standard are discussed in the following sections.

Protective Housing

A laser should have an enclosure around the laser that prevents access to radiant power or energy at levels *higher than the intended system classification.* A protective housing is required for all Class IIIa, IIIb, and IV lasers and an *interlock* must be provided on the protective housing of all Class IIIb and IV lasers that actuates on removal (or displacement) of the protective housing to prevent exposure to levels above the appropriate maximum permissible exposure (MPE) limits.

In some cases, a properly interlocked room (door interlocks, etc.) can be considered as the protective housing for an "open laser" provided that other engineering and/or procedural controls preclude operation at levels above those of the intended laser classification.

Key-Switch Interlocks

All Class IV lasers and laser systems shall have a key-switch master interlock. The key shall be removable and the laser shall not be capable of operation when the key is removed. Only authorized system operators shall have possession of the key. Inclusion of the key switch interlock on Class IIIb lasers and laser systems is also recommended for systems located in areas where nonauthorized medical personnel have nonsupervised access to the laser.

Interlocks should also be incorporated in conjunction with beam shutters when optical viewing systems such as telescopes or microscopes are used to view the beam or beam reflection area under potentially hazardous conditions. In this case, the interlock should prevent laser system operation when the beam shutter is removed from the optical system viewing path. Optical interlock systems are required for all Class III and IV laser systems.

Beam Path Enclosures

There are some uses of Class IIIb and IV lasers and laser systems where the entire beam path should be enclosed. This includes, for example, the area where the interaction of the primary or secondary beams occurs. It is recommended that such beam enclosures be equipped with appropriate safety interlocks to prevent operation unless the enclosures are properly installed and all means of operator access are secured.

Such a completely enclosed system, if properly safeguarded with interlocks so that all requirements for a Class I laser system are fulfilled, may be operated in the enclosed manner *without additional control measures.* Suitable controls for the enclosed laser classification are required (perhaps on a temporary basis) when the beam enclosures are removed.

Beam Stop or Attenuator

Class IIIa, IIIb, and IV lasers or laser systems should be provided with a permanently attached beam stop or attenuator that reduces the output emission to a level at or below the appropriate MPE level when the laser system is on "standby."

Visual or Audible Warning System

An audible tone or bell and/or visual warning (such as a flashing light) is recommended as an area control for Class IIIb and IV laser operation. Such warning devices are to be activated on system start-up and are to be uniquely identified with the laser operation. Verbal "countdown" commands are an acceptable audible warning if they are required by the standard operating procedures associated with the medical facilities. The warnings should be activated prior to laser emission.

Viewing-Options and Windows

All viewing portals, optics, windows, or display screens included as an integral part of an enclosed laser or laser installation shall incorporate some means to attenuate the laser radiation transmitted through the portal to levels below the appropriate MPE levels. This would include, for example, a "viewing window" into a clinic or operating room that serves as the system enclosure.

Interlock Requirements

Adjustments or procedures during service on the laser shall not cause the safety interlocks to become inoperative or the laser radiation outside a Class

I laser protective housing to exceed the MPE limits, unless a *temporary laser-controlled area* is established.

Interlocks for pulsed lasers or laser systems shall be designed so as to prevent laser operation when the interlock is closed by such methods as dumping stored capacitor-bank energy into a dummy load.

Interlocks for Class IIIb and IV continuous-wave or repetitively pulsed lasers shall, if closed, turn off the power supply or insert a shutter in the beam. Interlocks shall *not* allow re-energizing of the power supply when the interlock is closed.

All Class IIIb or IV lasers or laser systems should be provided with a remote interlock connector to allow electrical connections to an emergency master disconnect ("panic button") interlock or to room, door, or fixture interlocks.

Laser Controlled Area

When the entire beam path from a Class IIIb or IV laser is not sufficiently enclosed and/or baffled such that access to radiation above the MPE is possible, a "laser controlled area" shall be established. The following are requirements for such an area.

1. Have direct supervision of the laser safety officer (LSO) or his or her designee during all times of operation.

2. Required approved entry for any noninvolved personnel.

3. Be posted with appropriate warning signs.

4. Terminate all potentially hazardous beams.

5. Where appropriate, use diffusely reflecting materials near the beam (Class IIIb conditions only).

6. Incorporate appropriate safety interlocks at the doorways. Such latches shall, at all times, allow for egress by those in the laser-controlled area. (Class IV requirement only.) It should be noted that proposed revisions to the ANSI Z136 standard allow for other means (barriers, etc.) at entry ways to provide equivalent protection.

7. Authorized personnel may enter the area if there is no hazard at the entry point and if the appropriate eye protection is worn by the entering personnel. (Class IV requirement only.)

8. The beams shall not, under any circumstances, be allowed to be transmitted from the controlled area unless for specific atmospheric testing where the operator and the LSO assures that the beam path is limited to controlled air space.

Laser Warning Signs and Labels

Lasers and laser systems not bearing the laser warning logo shall be properly labeled in accordance with the ANSI Z136.1 standards as follows:

1. CAUTION: All signs and labels associated with Class II lasers. Also, all Class IIIa lasers with the special instruction: "Do not stare into beam or view directly with optical instruments."

2. DANGER: All signs and labels associated with Class IIIb and Class IV lasers and laser systems.

3. Class IIa lasers and laser systems require only a label that reads: "Laser Radiation—output not intended for viewing—avoid long-term viewing of the direct beam."

Area posting is required only for Class IIIb and Class IV lasers and laser systems.

Administrative and Procedural Controls

A written Standard Operating Procedure is required for Class IIIb and Class IV laser and laser systems.

The overall laser safety program is administered by the LSO. The principal responsibility is to establish and periodically review appropriate control measures, to avoid needless duplication of controls in cases where several alternate but equally effective means may be used to limit exposure, and to provide training.

Personal Protective Equipment

Personal protective equipment for laser safety generally means eye protection in the form of goggles or special prescription eyewear using special high-optical-density filter materials to reduce the potential ocular exposure below MPE limits. Some applications may dictate the use of a skin cover if long-term (repeated) exposures are anticipated at exposure levels at or near the MPE limits.

In general, it is recommended that, if possible, other means of controls be employed rather than reliance specifically on the use of protective eyewear. In the medical environment, this would apply to that equipment that is self contained, such as diagnostic systems.

A wide variety of commercially available optical filter glass (and plastics) are available for laser eye protection. Some are available in eye spectacles ground to prescription specifications. One filter-type may be applicable to more than one wavelength. Some filters have a high optical density below a certain "cutoff" wavelength, usually limiting overall visibility.

Special Control Measures

Infrared (700–10^6 nm) laser radiation and ultraviolet (200–400 nm) laser radiation are "invisible" radiation and require some special control measures:

Termination of Beam-Path.—The beams from Class IIIb and Class IV lasers should be terminated in highly absorbent, nonspecular reflecting materials wherever practicable. Note should be made that many metal surfaces that appear "dull" visually can act as a specular reflector of infrared radiation.

All secondary beams from reflections should be appropriately terminated in an absorbent material. Note: periodic inspection is required of the absorber materials since they degrade with use. Firebrick materials containing beryllium or other hazardous substances should not be used. An optical absorber wedge is recommended for beam termination.

Associated Hazards

Special attention shall be given to the possibility of producing undesirable reactions in the presence of ultraviolet radiation, for example, formation of skin sensitizing agents, ozone, etc.

BIBLIOGRAPHY

1. Rockwell R.J. (ed.): *Laser Safety in Surgery and Medicine,* ed. 2. Cincinnati, Ohio, Rockwell Associates, Inc., 1985.
2. Morgan K.Z.: Energy pollution of the environment, in *Electronic Product Radiation and the Health Physicist,* Proceedings of the Fourth Annual Mid-year Symposium, Health Physics Society. D.H.E.W. Publication No.: BRH/DEP 70–26, 1970, pp. 8–39.
3. Rockwell R.J.: Laser safety and training: Reviewing risks and safety protocols, and learning from case studies: How to avoid laser accidents, in Breedlove B., Schwartz D. (eds.): *Clinical Lasers: Expert Strategies for Practical and Profitable Management,* Part I. Atlanta, Ga., American Health Consultants, Inc., 1985.
4. American National Standard for the Safe Use of Lasers. No.: Z-136.1 (1980). New York, American National Standards Institute, 1980.
5. *Laser Safety Guide.* Laser Institute of America, Toledo, Ohio, 1985.
6. Rockwell R.J.: *Laser Safety Training Manual,* ed. 6. Cincinnati, OH., Rockwell Associates, Inc., 1984.

7. Rockwell R.J., Moss C.E.: Optical radiation hazards in laser welding processes, Part I: Neodymium—YAG laser. *J. Amer. Industrial Hygiene Assoc.* 44:572–579, 1983.
8. Schellhas H.F., Rockwell R.J.: Safety standards of the American National Standards Institute relevant to carbon dioxide laser surgery. *Proceedings of the Second International Congress on Gynecologic Laser Surgery.* Montreal, Canada, May, 1982.
9. Sliney D.H., Wolbarsht M.L.: *Safety With Lasers and Other Optical Sources.* New York, Plenum Press, 1980, pp. 65–185.
10. Rockwell R.J., Goldman L.: Research on human skin laser damage threshold, Final Report. University of Cincinnati, Contract F41609-72-C-0007, School of Aerospace Medicine, Brooks Air Force Base, Texas, 1972.
11. Goldman L., Rockwell R.J.: *Lasers in Medicine.* New York, Gordon & Breach Science Publishers, 1971.
12. Anderson R.R., Parrish J.A.: The optics of human skin, in Regan J.D., Parrish J.A. (eds.): *The Science of Photomedicine.* New York, Plenum Press, 1982.
13. Davis T.P.: The heating of skin by radiant energy, in Herzfeld C.M. (ed.): *Temperature, Its Measurement and Control in Science and Industry,* vol. 3, Part 3. New York, Reinhold Publishing Co., 1963, pp. 149–169.
14. Hayes J.R., Wolbarsht M.R.: Thermal model for retinal damage induced by pulsed lasers. *Aerospace Med.* 39:474–480, 1968.

3 Anesthesia Problems in Laser Surgery*

Martin L. Norton, M.D., J.D.

"The only merit I possess is that I know I know not."
Book of Proverbs

Anesthesiology has been in the forefront of medical-surgical progress from its inception as a physician specialty. Each development in surgical technology has meant a challenge to the anesthesiologist. The advent of laser surgery, particularly in its application to the aerodigestive tract, has provided the ultimate challenge in teamwork and airway management.

PREOPERATIVE PREPARATION

Problems of patient evaluation are compounded by the urgency of surgery in the patient whose airway is progressively occluded. Other medical conditions, usually mitigating against immediate surgery until alleviated, must be accepted and dealt with intraoperatively. The concept of teamwork becomes a critical reality rather than mere verbiage. Airway management is now crucial, and a joint cooperative endeavor of everyone—surgeon, anesthesiologist, and nursing staff. There are no delineated jobs—each person must help each and every other member of the team. It is imperative that the surgeon keep the anesthesiologist informed, in detail, of the specifics of the planned surgery. It is equally mandatory that the anesthesiologist understand and be supportive of the needs of the surgery and the patient.

Patients often present with airway obstructive disease. Even in cases where the lesion does not embarrass the airway, the anesthesiologist must

*Presented at the 1984 ENT Laser Congress held at Northwestern University Medical School in June, 1984.

recognize its potential in the anesthetized patient. Relaxation of pharyngeal and laryngeal supporting structures can convert a minimal lesion into a major obstructive situation. Medical conditions may ordinarily require delay of surgery (e.g., cardiac, diabetic, or other endocrine). Wherever possible, the patient should be treated to improve control of the disease. However, every member of the team must put the primary and complicating features in perspective. A clear airway is paramount. Other pathology falls into place in decreasing order of importance. Respiratory infections do not improve unless the airway is patent. Diabetic patients will not come under control unless concomitant infections are corrected. A good heart cannot function in the absence of available oxygen—and a bad cardiovascular system requires an optimal airway.

Fortunately for our purposes, the laser, of itself, produces minimal stress. In the aerodigestive system, the risk is mostly anesthesiologic. To be sure, complications can occur from use of the instrument. Electrical injuries related to grounding (e.g., burns) and interference with ECG and other monitors resulting in harm to the patient do occur. At this writing, a number of electrocutions have occurred among operators of laser instruments.[1] Surprisingly, knowledgeable individuals have been involved when they let their cautionary guard down. It is possible that the problem is related to the plasma phenomenon of magneto gas dynamics. A plasma is a fluid in which there are charged carriers, but which itself as a whole is electrically neutral, in the sense that the number of positive and negative charges are equal. The presence of the charged carriers renders the plasma electrically conductive and therein lies the risk of electrical injury. This is of even greater significance for patients with cardiac pacemakers or phrenic nerve stimulators. However, most situations involve basic principles of grounding and common sense precautions to be observed when handling high-voltage equipment.

We must not forget the anesthesiologist's responsibility to be constantly alert to electrical hazards. Improper grounding may result in burns at the sites of EGG lead attachments, and even in the area of the grounding pad attachment to the patient. Another risk relates to patients with implanted pacemakers. Floating grounds, intercouplers, and other isolation or run-off systems are available to cope with this problem.[2] They are prevented by the alert practitioner aware of the physics of the problem in patient application.

ENDOTRACHEAL TUBES

Anesthesia planning for equipment requires due deliberation. Even momentary failure can lead to disaster. Endotracheal tubes must be protected with precision. The alternative choice of Venturi ventilation requires due consideration of risks, advantages, and propriety of application. Instrumentation is every bit as important for the safe conduct of anesthesia management, as it is for surgical procedures. The laser can burn through into vital areas (e.g., superior mediastinum), cause a fire in the lumen of the laryngotrachea or bronchi. The anesthesiologist must be prepared for these, and a multitude of other medical problems. Preparation of drugs to be held in readiness of need, instrumentation available for potential use—these are among the keystones of safety. If red rubber endotracheal tubes are used, they must be carefully wrapped with reflective metal foil. No wrinkles, blisters, or gaps can be permitted. The foil must be applied smoothly, obliquely from the Murphy eye or cuff up the shaft of the tube as far as the exposed area of risk. The objective is to defract, scatter, or defocus the laser beam rather than reflect or focus it elsewhere, and to protect the underlying tube from heat intensity of a level to produce combustion. Wrapping of wired tubes (anode or armoured) does *not* permit their use, because of internal heating of the wire coil, resulting in melting of the internal lamina potentially obstructing the tube and blocking ventilation. Use of silicone tubes has been recommended (Milhaud, Xomed Laser Shield).[3] A more recent generation of the Milhaud tube requires use of nitrogen gas above the cuff to diminish combustibility and propagation of the flame from the hydrocarbon substrate when pure oxygen is used for artificial ventilation.*

Special comment and emphasis is required regarding the process of combustion. The misconception is that the sole key to the process is oxygen. In reality, the keystone is the "specific heat of combustion" factor (flash point) for the substrate. In our situation, it is the endotracheal tube, or the adhesive tape, or other substances exposed to the focused laser beam.[4] This is of particular note in view of the spate of purportedly "safe" endotracheal tubes for use with the laser (e.g., silicone tubes, etc.). Careful reading of the manufacturer's brochure (often ineptly reviewed by inexperienced products' liability attorneys), indicates "safety" at "atmospheric oxygen levels." In practice, we often use 100% oxygen levels, and always require greater than atmospheric 21% (at sea level) oxygen tensions. The safety of our patients requires a significant margin of safety in *all* equipment and techniques. No thorough studies have yet been done to evaluate effects of multigas systems under the stress of laser heat, i.e., nitrous oxide and other gas (halocarbons) dissociation phenomena based on pyrolysis reactions. At this writing, there are *no* totally safe endotracheal tubes other than possibly the Hirschman[5] and Norton[6] metal tubes; therefore we are we left with "relatively safe" red rubber, silicone base (not silicone coated) and the Milhaud (double gas concept) tubes.

*Milhaud nitrogen gas tube, Porges, Paris.

When we use the metal tubes, we often have to place a cuff to maintain a seal in the airway below the level of laser burn. This cuff *is* flammable. However, we can diminish the risk resulting from this potential by inflating the cuff and its pilot tube with a quenching liquid. At the moment the laser pierces the balloon cuff, the liquid leaks out, absorbing the heat and reducing the temperature at the ignition site. We prefer use of 1% aqueous lidocaine as the inflating medium. This choice seems optimal, since tissue reactivity to the momentary fire flare will be decreased by the local anesthetic effect.

The metal coil tubes are not airtight. The Norton tube was specifically designed to decrease the possibility of the endotracheal tube itself heating up and producing direct metal contact burns. The anesthetic system can readily compensate for this minimal leak by increased gas volume flows. Fortunately, the use of Venturi ventilation (according to the technique described herein) is available to aleviate the need for endotracheal tubes in most instances (see below). Similarly, the Woo-Sanders adapter (Pilling) to the Norton tube (V. Mueller) has filled the gap. The most obvious use of the Woo adapter, as applied to an uncuffed endotracheal tube, is in laser surgery of tracheal stenosis. This is the situation wherein avoidance of any intratracheal pressure is a major objective.

VENTURI VENTILATION

Venturi ventilation, first suggested by Sanders for bronchoscopic manipulation, comes to its peak in this era of the laser. This is based on the fact that light and gases can be transmitted along the same general pathway. Much has been written about Venturi ventilation.[7–9] The technique we recommend for laryngoscopic surgery utilizes a needle-on-clamp (Fig 3–1). This is relatively inexpensive, since it can be applied to almost any operating laryngoscope, and specifically to the Jako and Dedo laryngoscopes. The jet system includes a needle mounted on a clamp, a manual trigger, and a gauge and reducing valve. The injection needle must be made of stainless steel. Even microflecks of a chromium plated or aluminum needle can produce severe tissue reactivity in the lung field. When the needle is bent to fit conveniently on the clamp, the shaft must be annealed to prevent intraluminal crimping. Our preference for a manual trigger (adjusted to an all-or-none action) is based on continuing awareness of the ventilatory sequence. Automatic ventilator hypnosis (reliance) is usually based on the sound of the ventilator but does *not* assure adequacy of ventilation. Furthermore, it is often necessary to vary ventilatory patterns to meet the needs of the surgical procedure. As discussed previously,[10] we have used as little as 3 to 4

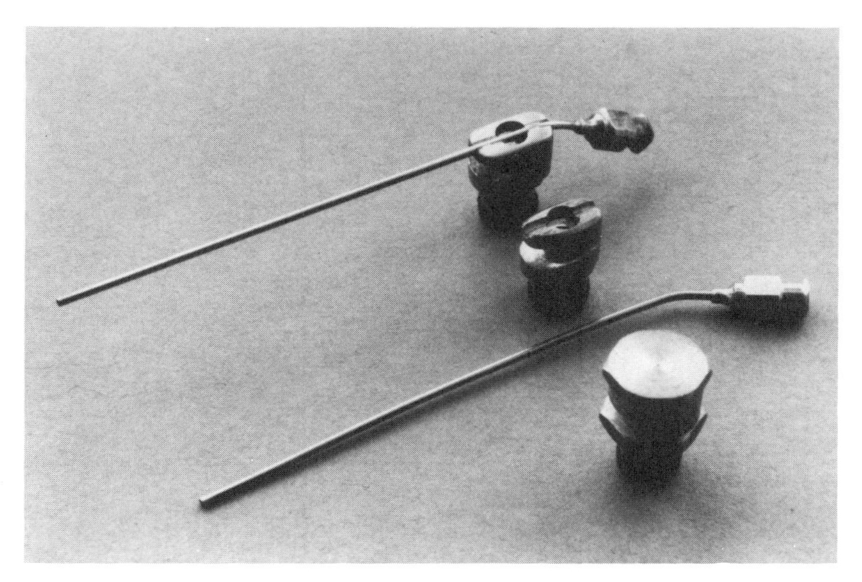

Fig 3–1. Venturi needle on clamp.

pounds per square inch (psi) for the pediatric patient, but rarely more than 40 to 45 psi for the relatively obese patient. In fact, we are concerned about the significant risk of pneumotrachea, pneumomediastinum, or even pneumothorax when using higher pressures. We also stress, most emphatically, that a break-away system of delivery tubing between the trigger and the patient should be used to avoid barotrauma. To further emphasize—high-pressure tubing should *never* be used on the patient side of the delivery tubing! When using the injector needle system attached to the proximal side of the laryngoscope, *continuous* suction through a side port must not be permitted, since it tends to suck out ventilatory gases from the lungs during the expiratory phase. Our continuing experience after thousands of cases cross-checked with arterial blood gases on a random basis indicates the efficacy of this technique. The advantage of this system is its applicability to almost any kind of laryngoscope, its minimal cost to produce the instrumentation, and *above all* the absolute absence of any tube or "pilot tube"[11,12] (as in the Carden tube or Injectoflex-Rusch)* in the airway.

Its disadvantages include drying of the laryngeal structures by the gas emitted from the jet as well as the movement of the vocal folds secondary to the force of the jet impinging thereon. This "disadvantage" is utilized in

*Injectoflex,® Willy Rusch, Rimelshausen, West Germany.

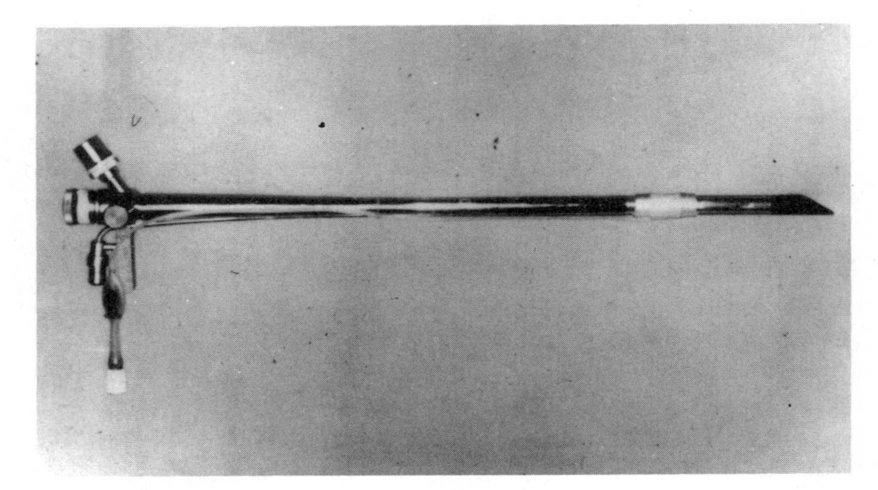

Fig 3–2. Cuffed bronchoscope, ventilating ports protected with metal tape.

another, nonlaser procedure—Teflon injection of the vocal fold. The sail-like filling of the vocal fold helps the surgeon judge the optimum movement of the folds and therefore the amount of Teflon to introduce into the paralyzed "cord." Another disadvantage is the risk of tissue dissection leading to pneumotrachea or pneumomediastinum if the jet is immediately used after a cold knife incision, as well as the risk of blowing blood into the tracheobronchial tract. If pneumotrachea, pneumomediastinum, or pneumothorax is suspected, complete radiologic studies should be immediately obtained to determine the magnitude of the problem. If the pneumoinjection is radiologically significant, and/or supported by aberration in the arterial blood gases, or accompanied by ECG changes, surgical insertion of appropriate drains is urgently required. Fortunately, the laser cut or burn usually seals the tissue, limiting the risks of pneumotrachea.

ENDOBRONCHIAL SURGERY

Prior to the advent of the laser, endobronchial surgery was limited to removal of foreign bodies and biopsy procedures. With development of the CO_2 laser, we then proceeded to palliative extirpation of intraluminal tumor masses via a specially adapted rigid ventilating bronchoscope.[13] The obvious problem is, how do you ventilate both lungs while permitting the endoscopist to accomplish his surgical objective? We did this in a rudimentary fashion with a cuffed bronchoscope (Fig 3–2) intermittently inserting it into the bronchi, then withdrawing it above the carina. The development of the Nd:YAG laser transmitted via fiberoptics opened a new parameter for intraluminal surgery. However, it does *not* alleviate the problem of patient ventilation. We are now faced with four choices.

One technique involves use of the fiberoptic instrument in the awake, spontaneously ventilating patient under local anesthesia. The risk here is that the patient may cough, move, or retch. The operator is then working on a moving target with risk of burning undesired areas.

The second approach is use of an anesthetic technique and placement of a small lumen endotracheal tube for ventilation and insertion of the fiberoptic laser instrument alongside. The problem now to be faced is the difficulty in maintaining a leakproof airway.

The third approach is analogous to fiberoptic bronchoscopy under general anesthesia in the intubated patient through a Portex® swivel adapter (Fig 3–3). This would be the ideal solution, assuming that the diameter of the fiberoptic laser instrument passed through the endotracheal tube still provides for adequate passage of gases (anesthetic, O_2 or CO_2) (Fig 3–4). The fourth approach, and most current, is the return to our rigid bronchoscope technique—passing the laser fiber intraluminally under direct vision. This approach is best conducted using the Sanders' technique of ventilation, or use of the Wolf-Dumon ventilating bronchoscope.

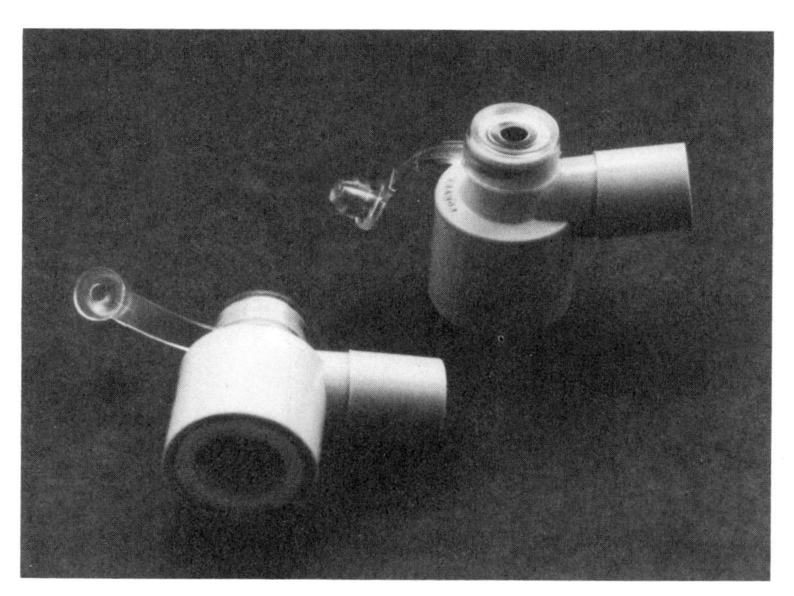

Fig 3–3. Portex® swivel adapter.

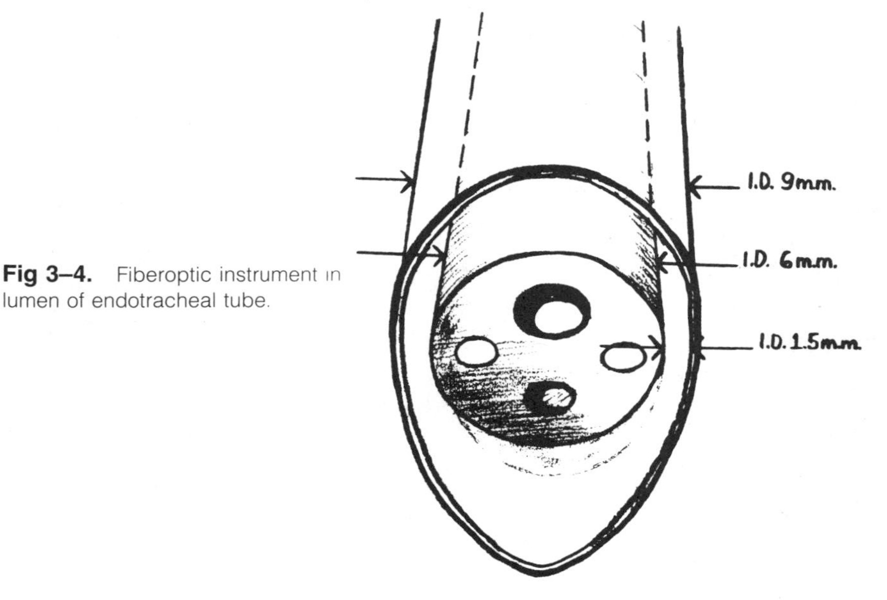

Fig 3–4. Fiberoptic instrument in lumen of endotracheal tube.

TRACHEOTOMIZED PATIENT MANAGEMENT

The patient with a tracheotomy can be managed relatively easily. Use of the ventilating rigid bronchoscope with superposed lidocaine inflated cuff has been discussed above. Another option is the Sanders-Venturi technique* without a cuff, but this would obviate attachment of the operating microscope to the optic end of the bronchoscope. We prefer to insert a cuffed metal tracheotomy tube or Norton tube, pack wet patti-pads cephalad to this cuff, and proceed with the laryngeal laser surgery. There is no reason to risk metal foil wrapping of plastic tubes.

TUBE WRAPPING

Recently, it has come to our attention that the previously recommended Radio Shack® sensor tape, as well as some 3M® sensor tape recommended for alternate reflective wrapping of red rubber endotracheal tubes, has been changed in its reflective properties. Since *no* reflective tape is specifically manufactured for laser tube wrapping, it is incumbent on the user to check and constantly recheck, with the laser beam, the reflective properties of the

*Xomed® Laser-Shield Endotracheal Tube, Cuffed. Jacksonville, Fla., 32216.

tape. We have abandoned use of the Radio Shack® sensor tape and occasionally use one-quarter in. to one-half in. 3M tape *after thorough and repeated* checking.* (The medicolegal implications of using a reflective tape not approved by the FDA for human use is mentioned but not discussed herein.)

MANAGEMENT OF A LASER FIRE

What *do* we do for management of laser-ignited intratracheal fire?[14] We have already commented on the preintubation lubrication of the larynx with lidocaine, and the need to keep the area around the burn wet. When combustion takes place, the laser is discontinued and the area of conflagration must be quenched with water. (We keep an Asepto® syringe filled with water immediately available with the surgical instruments.)

Another approach utilizes the experience of fuel chemists and physicists, to wit: The Venturi system involves compressing a gas under pressure. When the gas leaves the egress port it expands. Expansion is accompanied by a marked decrease in temperature. This temperature drop is communicated by the properly directed jet to the base of the flame, and the combustible hydrocarbon (e.g., endotracheal tube or patti-pad). By reducing the temperature below the "flash point," the fire will be extinguished.

Immediate removal of the combustible substrate (endotracheal tube), followed by a lidocaine spray flush, is highly recommended. This, however, assumes that reintubation with a siliconized tube presents no problem. There are other circumstances wherein the mechanics of intubation are such that removal of a still patent tube might present a major risk, especially in view of the postcombustion edema, from the burn. At that point, a Norton stylet (Teflon or silicone, Fig 3–5) should be introduced through the endotracheal tube and the burned tube removed over the stylet. Next a fresh, *uncuffed* silicone tube should be threaded over the stylet into the trachea to maintain the airway during the posttrauma period of acute edema and potential airway closure. The patient should receive ultrasonic humidification of the area around the silicone tube and of the tracheobronchial tree. An intravenous stress dose of Solumedrol,® type-specific antibiotics, and systemic support of the respiration follows. Of great importance is monitoring with arterial blood gas studies and end-tidal P_{CO_2} studies to guide further respiratory therapy. The ventilatory quotient (utilizing the concept of the A-a difference to determine respiratory management) is crucial to therapy. In the event the above technique cannot be used, and assuming that diag-

*Minnesota Mining and Manufacturing, St. Paul, Minn. (3M No. 425).

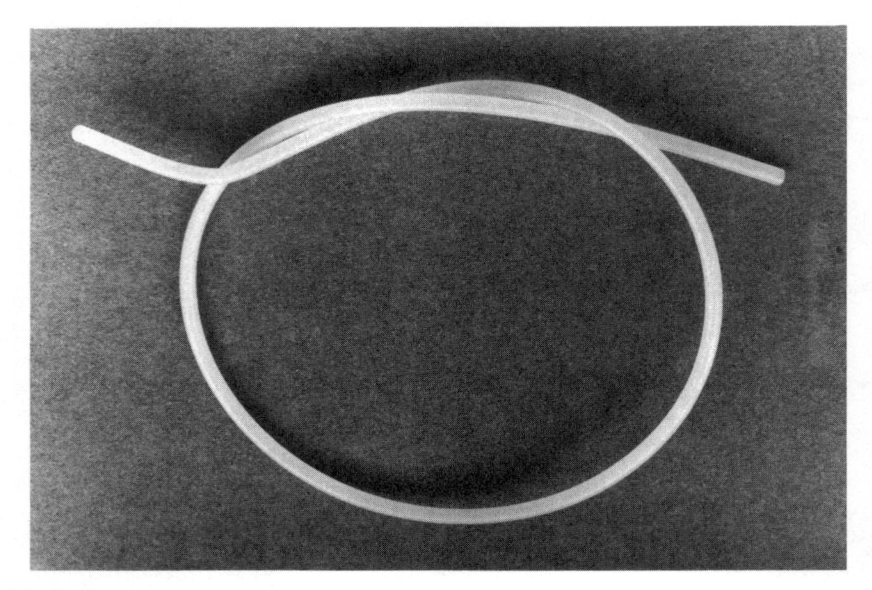

Fig 3–5. Norton teflon stylet.

nostic bronchoscopy indicates a severe burn of the laryngotracheobronchial tree, an immediate tracheotomy is required with insertion of a siliconized tracheotomy tube. The remainder of the therapy is determined by the patient's symptomatology and laboratory findings.

A question has been raised relative to risks of jet transfer of tissue particles and subsequent implantations in the tracheobronchial tree. To date, no evidence of any kind suggests that this tissue culture concept occurs. In fact, at the temperature of the spot-focused laser beam, the probability is that such debris or smoke is *nonvital* and that viruses, fungi, and the like would be killed. However, much needs to be done to evaluate these theoretic considerations.

Patient protection includes wet eye patches, use of canvas tape, constant concern for fire and stray laser radiation or reflection, as well as problems of pneumothorax and insufficient ventilation. Currently, we have initiated a consideration of the pyrolysis reactions of anesthetic gases to determine release and quantitation of breakdown products or polymerization reactions.[15] This was brought to our attention after inadvertent use of the laser on methylmethacrylate. The products of pyrolysis-releasing toxic substances such as phosgene, acrolein, and acrylic acid, among others, raised the question of pyrolysis reactions of inhalation anesthetics in general, and of the halogenated hydrocarbons in particular. In the interim, we urge consideration of IV anesthetic techniques to avoid the theoretic potential risks of pyrolytic breakdown or polymerization products of the anesthetic agents in the respiratory tract. This, however, must be balanced against the often observed hypertension placing the older and cardiac patient at risk[18] and for which the inhalation agents may be the drugs of choice.

OCULAR INJURY

Injury to the eyes is not limited to laser surgery.[16] What makes this topic important is the risk of direct or indirect (scatter or reflective) burns of the cornea. Direct focused radiation with the CO_2 laser would produce irreparable damage to the eye, involving the cornea and retina. Scatter radiation usually produces superficial damage to the cornea, conjunctiva, or eyelids. The key is related to the degree the columnated focused laser beam is broken up into its parts, i.e., defocused. With surgical instruments this may be accomplished by matte finishing the metal. Matte finishing of metal can be done by bombarding the metal with fine metal shot to pit the metal. Since we cannot be assured that any specific instrument is so properly treated, protection of the eyes should be done with wet eye pads held on with canvas tape and further assured by covering with wet cloth drapes *kept wet*. The reason for the moisture is based on its absorption properties for heat. Wet canvas (porous) retains the moisture so that incidental laser (heat) beams would *char* rather than produce combustion of the tape. Plastic or paper tape must be absolutely avoided because, like ointments and jellies, it tends to explode or flare up when exposed to the laser beam.

Protection of the eyes is also the keynote for persons working with the laser. We generally accept the concept that laser-specific protective glasses should be used by personnel in the room, but do not seem to recognize that most exposures are from scatter radiation. The positioning of scrub nurse, anesthesiologists, and circulator would more likely lead to scatter radiation crossing the cornea from the side—thus optic side guards are mandatory. The operating surgeon need not wear glasses, since he or she is usually protected by the operating microscope's lenses.

It is interesting to note[17] that with the recommended procedures very few eye injuries have been reported. This speaks for the conclusion that awareness of hazards coupled with preventive measures *can* serve to mitigate the risk. However, the risk is still there, as indicated by the records of the Bureau of Radiologic Health, Radiation Incidents Registry.[18]

The ease and apparent simplicity of laser application and Venturi ventilation belie the real and potential hazards. Laser hypnosis plagues the surgeon just as ventilation automaticity can fool the anesthesiologist.

LASER SURGERY IN THE DIGESTIVE TRACT

The major concerns here relate to intraluminal gases and the ease of perforation of the digestive tract at the site of pathology. In the event of inadvertent perforation of the digestive tract, the anesthesiologist must be ready for management of an immediate thoracotomy or laparotomy. This implies major surgicoanesthetic preparation for each case.

The second hazard is related to combustion of the gases in the digestive tract (including methane). The combustion is usually very rapid and therefore in the nature of an explosion. A slower rate of combustion would result in an intraluminal fire. Here, again, the anesthesiologist must be prepared for opening the chest or abdomen.

ANESTHETIC AGENTS AND ADJUVANTS

It is self-evident that we must avoid flammable anesthetic agents (e.g., the ethers).

Laryngoscopy may lead to tachycardia, hypertension, and myocardial ischemia. Strong et al.[19] found an increased incidence of myocardial ischemia and infarct following suspension laryngoscopy. This often requires vasodilators, beta blockers, and/or deeper anesthetic levels. Indeed, potent inhalation agents can be carefully titrated and are highly effective in blunting the hemodynamic responses to laryngoscopy and intubation. Fentanyl (8 to 10 mg/kg) along with thiopental sodium or nitrous oxide, similarly blunt heart rate and pressure responses to intubation. Intravenous lidocaine (1.5 mg/kg) or intratracheal lidocaine (160 mg) slightly reduces heart rate increases while reducing blood pressure (BP) changes.[20, 21] We prefer use of Innovar, a combination of a short-acting narcotic (fentanyl) and a long-acting ganglionic blocker (droperidol). Innovar is an excellent premedicant in the unobstructed patient. Lorazepam would approach the ideal preanesthetic agent were it not for its long action. This drug also produces antegrade amnesia.[22, 23] We do prefer Innovar, however, because of its antihypertensive action (antagonizing the epinephrine-induced hypertension produced during suspension laryngoscopy).

We recommend the use of a lidocaine spray (1%) before intubation, and after extubation. Our objective is multifold: (a) to lubricate the area surrounding the intended burn site and (b) to provide a modicum of anesthetic effect and reduce the reactivity of burned tissue thereby diminishing the potential postinjury fibrosis, and lastly (c) to decrease the incidence of postanesthesia laryngospasm.

Another consideration is the choice of muscle relaxants. We prefer succinylcholine IV titration. This is a short-acting agent requiring no antagonist after short cases. While we find no contraindications to pancuronium chloride (curare group), they often need reversal at the close of surgery. The reversal agents classically include a belladonna and prostigmine. Both of these drugs tend to increase the viscosity of secretions. The problem, however hypothetical, relates primarily to surgery in the anterior commissure or the anterior one third of the vocal cords. The laser produces a raw-heated tissue residuum. Venturi ventilation tends to dry the same tissues. Thus we have the ideal potential for approximation of the raw dry surfaces, their cohesion by capillary action, and at least a realistic potential for developing an anterior commissure web. We avoid this by use of an IV succinyldiacetylcholine drip. A new agent, atracurium, recently introduced, has to be evaluated in this context.

Monitoring the patient is the safety factor anesthesiologists have always dealt with. Ascertaining ventilatory adequacy is an obligation of the anesthesiologist. This is also a prime consideration of monitoring, which, when coupled with cardiovascular parameters, indicates to a great extent the viability of the patient. Arterial blood gas studies are the best guides to ventilatory parameters and electrolyte balances. The precordial stethoscope, when combined with BP measurements and the patterns reflected in the ECG, are most frequently used to reflect cardiovascular status. The additions of measurements obtained from the arterial pressure and blood gas specimens, and Swan-Ganz catheter, including cardiac output studies, completes the state of the art for understanding of cardiorespiratory function.

While using the Venturi, we note particularly the movement of the thoracic cage. Our experience has repeatedly demonstrated a direct correlation between the thoracic excursion and adequacy of the arterial blood levels relative to oxygenation and CO_2 levels in the usual patient. Despite this, we still randomly review arterial blood gases during anesthetic management.

EXTUBATION: THE END OF SURGERY AND ANESTHESIA

"To do or not to do, that is the question?"

The major question at the end of surgery in the aerodigestive tract is: "How do we manage the airway in the immediate postoperative period?". The answer involves a complexity of considerations. The obese patient is the "plus perfect" example of this group. We must consider the energy requirement of respiratory effort, the need for additional tissue perfusion, and the positioning of the larynx in relation to the root of the tongue. These are only a few of the factors suggesting a tendency to airway obstruction. Some other factors include micrognathia, temporomandibular joint disease, atlanto-axial instability, Marie-Strumpel arthritis of the neck, acromegaly, craniofacial dysostosis, and infiltrations of the tongue. The patient who has had esophageal instrumentation often awakens with a choking sensation similar to a classic dyspnea. This is the residuum of the instrument in the esophagus and may include an element of intrusion against the soft posterior wall of the trachea. We like to keep the endotracheal tube in situ until the patient is assuredly alert enough to breath adequately and also can be in communication for reassurance. It seems to us that patients tolerate removal of the endotracheal tube much earlier after bronchoscopy than after esophagoscopic manipulation.

With regard to laser surgery of the trachea and bronchi, the earlier an endotracheal tube is removed (foreign-body reaction), the better. We must always be cognizant of the risk of tracheal stenosis, whether it is due to mucosal ischemia produced by an inflated indwelling endotracheal tube or secondary to fibrotic reaction following laser surgery and edema deposition.

However, laser surgery of the larynx is not quite as easy as the above. If the surgery is done under Venturi ventilation, we prefer *not* to reintubate and potentially irritate the laryngeal structures. This option may not be afforded us if the surgery was extensive and particularly if significant edema ensues. In the latter situation it may be wiser to insert a small siliconized plastic tube until the patient is fully alert and the immediate period of full edema has passed. Hopefully, this time period would have been self limited by use of corticoid therapy and the lidocaine spray. There are no specific studies demonstrating beneficial effects of corticosteroids during laser surgery management. The basis for corticoid use is by extrapolation from extensive studies of steroid effects on inflammation.[24] Histopathologic changes adjacent to the laser burn are close analogues to inflammatory pathology and justify corticosteroid use to reduce edema and fibrosis. In adults, we use 4 mg of dexamethasone before laser use and repeat this before leaving the operating theater and again in the recovery room.

The decision to extubate, or to reintubate can only be made at the end of the procedure and requires a bit of professional maturity, and a whole lot of judgment (sometimes synonymous with luck).

At *all* times, the equipment and the facility to intubate the patient postoperatively must be available. Fortunately, most patients pass the critical time frame within one hour postoperatively.

Another aid is the position of the patient. Reference to the superb books by Fink,[25] and Fink and Demarest[26] will remind the reader of the spring-coil mechanism of the larynx and its suspensory structures. Sitting the patient up opens the internal diameters of the larynx and tracheobronchial tree to its maximum, and permits optimum lymphatic drainage. The biomechanics of ventilation is thus aided (including the diaphragmatic excursion).

Last, the patient should have ultrasonic water nebulization (0.5 or less) for a minimum period of two hours following surgery. Larger size particles merely coalesce and run down into the tracheobronchial tree. Also, some patients seem to be more comfortable with an ice collar for the first hour. Whether this is a physiologic or a psychologic response does not matter if the patient is calmer and breathes more rhythmically and quietly.

THE ARGON LASER

This medium has become of some interest in the field of otolaryngology.[27,28] It emits blue-greenish light with its energy being preferentially absorbed by objects in the red spectrum. A major advantage is its transmissibility along fiberoptic bundles and its focusability to a very small impact point. Some consideration has been given as to its use in stapes surgery.[29] A possible disadvantage in its use elsewhere is related to its fine pinpoint focus requiring multiple impacts or burns. This is primarily a time-of-application factor. However, it also relates to depth of the burn following multiple impacts at the same site and potential perforation. At the present time this mode of therapy is still being studied. However, its use in debulking and removal of acoustic neuromas, mucosal telangiectasias, hemangiomas, and cystic hygromas show great promise. Use of the argon laser for laryngeal papillomas is a tedious process, possibly causing more scar formation. The use of this laser medium has presented no unique anesthesiologic problems. Principles of anesthetic management discussed herein apply with equal import.

No discussion of problems and complications would be complete without a discussion of standards for laser surgery. As in other areas of endeavor, the professional competency on which patients rely requires a process of learning, credentialing by the supervising institution, operational standards within the institution, and monitoring of this process. Organizations such as the American National Standards Institute (ANSI), the FDA, and the Occupational Safety and Health Administration are addressing these concerns with one view—the safety of the patient. While not discussing this aspect herein, we do append the standards initiated by the Laser Safety Committee of the University of Michigan (see Appendix A).

Last, and by no means least, in our litigious society, is the legal issue. An informed consent means more than just risks of the procedure. It means the moral and ethical acceptance of responsibility and the seeking to perfect one's knowledge and skills. Informed consent as a concept requires the physician to discuss the anesthetic management plans, alternatives, and potential complications of each. Implicit in this is communication of the experience of the physician with the technique. What is "routine" for one practitioner may be "experimental" for another.[30] It fact, the very integrity of the physician is at stake, as is the patient-physician relationship. Preparation of the professional for the privilege and honor of serving the patient (standard of care) is a burden we bear with due consideration of societal pressures.

This presentation has discussed not only the problems, but approached the solutions. We strive to point the way to providing the surgeon with conditions optimized for the benefit and safety of the patient. How well we have achieved this objective can only be determined by the success of the reader's efforts in behalf of and with safety for the patient.

REFERENCES

1. Franks J.K., Sliney D.H.: Electrical hazards of lasers. Electrooptical Systems Design, Dec. 1975, pp. 20–24.
2. Morrison R.: *Grounding and Shielding Techniques in Instrumentation,* ed 2. New York, John Wiley & Sons, 1977.
3. Milhaud A., Voquette G., Strobinsky E., et al.: Sonde d'intubation en silicone pour l'anesthesie generale en microchirurgie du larynx por le laser au CO_2. *Cashiers D'anesthesiologie* 27:717–720, 1979.
4. Burgess G.E., LeJeune F.E.: Endotracheal tube ignition during laser surgery of the larynx. *Arch. Otolaryngol.* 105:561–562, 1979.
5. Porch D., Hirschman C., Leon D., et al: Improved metal endotracheal tube for laser surgery of the airway. *Anesth. Analg.* 59:789–791, 1980.
6. Norton M.L., de Vos P.: A new endotracheal tube for laser surgery of the larynx. *Ann. Otol. Rhinol. Laryngol.* 87:554–558, 1978.
7. Spoerel W.E., Greenway R.E.: Technique of ventilation during endolaryngeal surgery under general anesthesia. *Can. Anaesth. Soc. J.* 20:369–377, 1973.
8. Sanders R.D.: Two ventilating attachments for bronchoscopes. *Del. Med. J.* 39(7):170–176, 1967.
9. Woo P., Eurenius S.: Dynamics of Venturi jet ventilation through the operating laryngoscope. *Ann. Otol. Rhinol. Laryngol.* 91:615–621, 1982.
10. Norton M.L., Strong M.S., Vaughan C.W., et al.: Endotracheal intubation and Venturi (jet) ventilation for laser microsurgery of the larynx. *Ann. Otol. Rhinol. Laryngol.* 85(5):656–664, 1976.
11. Carden E., Ferguson B.G.: A new technique for micro-laryngeal surgery in infants. *Laryngoscope* 83:691, 1973.
12. Carden E., Vest H.R.: Further advances in anesthetic techniques for microlaryngeal surgery. *Anesth. Analg.* 53:584, 1974.

13. Shapshay S.M., Davis R.K., Vaughn C.W., et al.: Palliation of airway obstruction from tracheobronchial malignancy: Use of the CO_2 laser bronchoscope. *Otolaryngol. Head Neck Surg.* 91:615–619, 1983.
14. Schramm V.L. Jr., Mattox D.E., Stool S.E.: Acute management of laser ignited intratracheal explosion. *Laryngoscope* 91:1417–1426, 1981.
15. Kroll D.A., Morris M., Norton M.L.: Pyrolysis products of halocarbons, work in progress, 1984.
16. Injury to eyes (industrial laser data references. American National Standards Institute and Rockwell Corporation).
17. Fried M.P.: A survey of the complications of laser laryngoscopy. *Arch. Otolaryngol.* 110:31–34, 1984.
18. Bureau of Radiologic Health, Radiation Incidents Registry, Food and Drug Administration, U.S. Department of Health and Human Services.
19. Strong M.S., Vaughan C.W., Mahler D.L., et al.: Cardiac complications of microsurgery of the larynx: Etiology, incidence and prevention. *Laryngoscope* 84:908–920, 1974.
20. Denhinger J.K., Ellison N., Ominsky A.G.: Effects of intratracheal lidocaine on circulatory responses to tracheal intubation. *Anesthesiology* 4:409, 1974.
21. Stoeling R.K.: Blood pressure and heart rate changes during short-duration laryngoscopy for tracheal intubation: influence of viscous or intravenous lidocaine. *Anesth. Analg.* 57:197, 1978.
22. Pandit S.K., Heisterkamp D.V., Cohen P.J.: Further studies of the anti-recall effect of lorazepam: A dose-time-effect relationship. *Anesthesiology* 45:495–500, 1976.
23. Kothary S.P., Brown A.C.D., Pandit U.A., et al.: Time course of antirecall effect of diazepam and lorazepam following oral administration. *Anesthesiology* 55:641–644, 1981.
24. Hawkins D.B., Crockett D.M., Shum T.K.: Corticosteroids in airway management. *Otolaryngol. Head Neck Surg.* 91:593–596, 1983.
25. Fink B.R.: *The Human Larynx.* New York, Raven Press, 1975.
26. Fink B.R., Demarest R.J.: *Laryngeal Biomechanics.* Cambridge, Mass. Harvard University Press, 1978.
27. Wilpizeski C.: Experimental labyrinthotomy in monkeys by argon and carbon dioxide lasers. *Otol. Head Neck Surg.* 89:197–203, 1981.
28. Williams D.J., Mitchell D.P.: The laser and the nasal septum: A histological study. *J. Otolaryngol.* 9:12, 1980.
29. Perkins R.C.: Laser stapedotomy for otosclerosis. *Laryngoscope* 90:228–241, 1980.
30. Norton M.L.: When does an experimental innovative procedure become an accepted procedure? *Pharos* 34:161–165, 1975.

4 Complications of Endoscopy and Their Prevention

James H. Kelly, M.D.

When a surgeon plans to do a "laser" procedure through an endoscope, it is easy to focus attention on the laser aspect of the procedure and fail to focus enough attention on the endoscopy itself. Complications have occurred with endoscopy long before the laser was invented, and while the use of the laser poses some unique problems, it does not remove the potential for endoscopic complications. Indeed, the amount of exposure necessary for a laser procedure may increase this risk.

Prevention of these complications requires attention to detail. This does not begin in the OR but rather at the initial assessment of the patient.

PREOPERATIVE ASSESSMENT

General Physical Condition.—A thorough assessment of the general physical condition of the patient should be undertaken. Particular attention should be paid to the status of the patient's airway and whether it can be maintained when the patient is under general anesthesia. If there is serious question of this, consideration should be given to a tracheotomy under local anesthesia prior to endoscopy. Pulmonary function and cardiac status should also be assessed carefully and appropriate measures taken to treat any underlying disorder. Medications that might affect the procedure should be noted.

A thorough history should be taken in regard to bleeding disorders, including use of aspirin and other medications that might affect clotting. Even small amounts of blood in the airway can cause laryngospasm. Any question of a bleeding problem should be investigated. A good screening test battery for bleeding problems should consist of a complete blood cell count (CBC), platelet count, prothrombin time, partial thromboplastic time, and bleeding time.

Metabolic disorders such as diabetes and thyroid disease should be identified by history, physical examination, and appropriate laboratory tests and treatment instituted where necessary. In summary, a thorough general physical assessment should be undertaken with particular emphasis on the airway and bleeding disorders.

In addition to this general physical assessment, certain problems such as described below, should be noted specifically, since, if they are severe enough, they might seriously alter or cancel an endoscopic procedure.

Neck Problems.—Conditions such as arthritis or prior cervical fusion that prevent extension of the neck indicate that exposure at endoscopy will be difficult, if not impossible, using a rigid endoscope. Scar contractures of the neck from burns or prior surgery can also prevent neck extension. Patients with significant arthritis of the cervical spine should be evaluated with an extension film of the neck. Similarly, patients with osteoporosis should be assessed to determine if the marked extension required in rigid endoscopy will produce excessive manipulation to the cervical spine.

Mandibular-Oropharyngeal Problems.—Patients with trismus, macroglossia, retrognathia, or microstomia can make rigid endoscopy difficult if not impossible. Since larger endoscopes are used with laser endoscopy, this must be taken into account in the evaluation. In some patients, the problem is so severe that a different approach must be used (such as endoscopic removal of a lesion without the laser permitting a smaller scope, or an external approach).

Condition of Teeth, Gums, Dentures.—Loose teeth, severe decay, gingival disease, and dentures and appliances that are fragile should be noted in the preoperative assessment. If possible, these problems should be corrected prior to endoscopy. If not enough time is available, these should be noted and the patient should be informed that damage could occur or that dentures or teeth could be dislodged, producing a foreign body in the airway and requiring removal.

Lesions of the Upper Aerodigestive Tract.—Careful assessment of all lesions should be noted and a description (preferably a picture) should be recorded. Friability or vascularity should also be noted. These observations should then be discussed with the anesthesiologist to determine the best method for intubation, etc. At this point a decision should be made as to whether intubation, Venturi inhalation, or tracheotomy would be safest for the patient. This decision should not have to be made during the operative procedure except in rare instances.

PREOPERATIVE MEDICATIONS

Careful discussion with anesthesia and/or medical consultants should determine which of the patient's ongoing medications should be continued and in what dosages. Heavy preoperative sedation should be avoided in patients with airway compromise. For further detailed information, see chapter 3.

INFORMED CONSENT

Informed consent will be discussed in another chapter in some detail; however, careful communication with the patient and/or family is necessary. Risks, benefits, and alternatives should be given and ample opportunity should be provided for questions. Printed material explaining the procedure and complications as well as postoperative expectations is quite helpful. This should be given to the patient as soon as possible so that it can be read over at the patient's leisure and questions formulated.

COMMUNICATIONS WITH OTHER PERSONNEL

All members of the team involved in the care of the patient, including anesthesiologists, floor and operating nurses, other physicians (residents, assistants, consultants), and, if necessary, workers in social services and nutrition, should understand the patient's problem as it pertains to their area. It is the surgeon's responsibility to inform these vital personnel of any particular problem that might occur relating to their area. Specialized equipment and medications should be ordered well in advance. Floor nurses should be made aware of the patient's problems and anticipated treatment so they can assist in preoperative and postoperative teaching. An accurate assessment of the amount of time a procedure should take is helpful in determining the choice of agents and in assigning of personnel.

Any failure of the surgeon to communicate to these other vital members of the team can result in a complication, an unhappy patient, or both.

OR

Careful Assessment of Equipment.—Prior to the procedure, the surgeon should assure himself that all necessary equipment is available and in working order. This is aided by a complete and precise surgeon's card and by pictures showing the equipment and room layout (see chapter 11 on "Nursing Aspects"). The positioning of the equipment should be well worked out prior to attempting the procedure. This will avoid a cluttered room and avoid injury to OR personnel. Thorough inservice sessions with OR personnel will help to assure a smoothly functioning room.

Positioning of the Patient.—Careful positioning of the patient on the OR table will allow good exposure during endoscopy and prevent injuries. As with all procedures, pressure points should be padded. In the tall patient, a table extension may be necessary to prevent the feet from hanging off. All OR personnel should be aware of the need for appropriate positioning in order to prevent abrasions and nerve palsies. It is obvious that the patient should be secured on the table with belts. For endoscopy, the patient should be positioned as shown in Figure 4–1. If anatomical or medical problems prevent this ideal position, it should be modified.

Protection of Eyes From Abrasion.—Prior to draping, the patient's eyes should be protected by the use of ophthalmic ointment. The eyes should then be taped shut using a nonallergic adhesive tape. This will prevent injury by abrasion from the drapes or by instruments. Eyes should be untaped and checked by the surgeon after the procedure.

Protection of Teeth and Gums.—After induction of general anesthesia and prior to the insertion of the endoscope, the teeth or gums should be protected using a tooth guard, or, if the patient is edentulous, a moist, folded gauze sponge. This should be checked after the endoscope is inserted and during the procedure to ensure that it has not been displaced. Teeth and gums should be inspected before and after insertion of the endoscope. Damage should be noted. Dislodged teeth or appliances should be found prior to leaving the OR. This may, at times, require further endoscopy and/or x-rays.

Exposure.—To assure adequate exposure, a large laryngoscope that allows binocular microscopic views of the aerodigestive tract must be used. For most instances, a Dedo-Pilling modified anterior commissure laryngoscope is satisfactory. The bronchoscope (with laser attachment) is also used

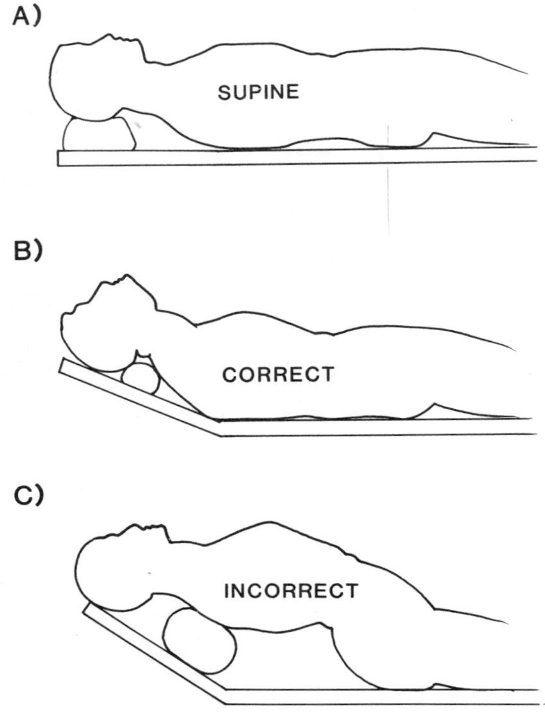

Fig 4–1. Diagram showing **A,** patient in supine position with head supported; **B,** correct positioning with roll under back and head extended, and **C,** incorrect positioning of patient with roll too far under back and head not fully extended.

in as large a size as the airway will permit. Larger scopes will also allow more maneuverability of instruments inserted through the scope. Good suction is necessary to remove blood and secretions. A vented, finger-controlled suction is best, since it avoids suctioning mucosa and subsequent damage.

Orderly Assessment of Aerodigestive Tract.—To prevent missing secondary lesions, an orderly assessment of the aerodigestive tract should be performed prior to any definitive tissue removal. This will avoid blood that will obscure the view. Vocal cord mobility, if not already assessed, should also be noted. This might require reversal of paralysis. If this assessment is necessary, the anesthesiologist should be consulted prior to the procedure as to timing and paralytic agents to be used.

Suspension System—Handling of Equipment.—To avoid unnecessary pressure during endoscopy, a suspension system should be used that produces a force vector in the direction shown in Figure 4–2 and that does not twist the endoscope. The Lewey system is simple to operate and is satisfactory for most procedures. It should be remembered that all endoscopes are "suspended" even though mechanical systems are not used. The length of most rigid endoscopes produces a degree of mechanical advantage due to the lever action that can cause considerable damage even with small motion. Rapid advancement of the scope or other instruments should be avoided. Adequate relaxation or paralysis is necessary during the procedure to prevent patient movement and injury. Proper size selection of the endoscope will also reduce the risk of injury (see above). Minimal pressure should be used to maneuver the endoscopes.

Faulty equipment can also cause injury by breaking or working in an improper manner. Likewise, the selection of the wrong instrument for the

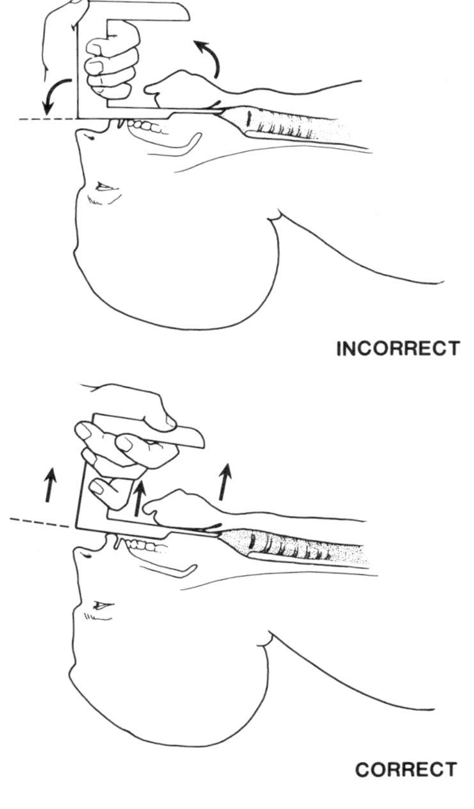

Fig 4–2. Incorrect vector for gaining exposure during laryngoscopy (note: pressure on teeth, upper lip) *(top.)* Correct vector to gain exposure during laryngoscopy (note: lift is straight rather than torquing laryngoscope) *(bottom).*

procedure can also produce damage (i.e., too delicate a forceps for removal of tough tissue can result in breakage of the instrument or tearing of normal structures).

Sharp instruments (knives, scissors) should be kept in optimal condition and handed carefully back to the scrub nurse. In no instance should they be left on the field or in an endoscope when not being used.

CAREFUL "MAPPING" OF BIOPSY SPECIMEN

Improper "mapping" or labeling of biopsy specimens can result in improper diagnosis and in an improper procedure. Numbered specimens, corresponding to a picture, should be carefully done and placed in separate, well-labeled containers. If possible, direct communication with the pathologist who is to examine the specimen is ideal. Tumor diagraming should be performed.

POSTOPERATIVE INTUBATION VS. TRACHEOTOMY

At the end of the procedure, the surgeon should reassess the airway to determine if swelling, blood, secretions, etc., will compromise ventilation in the postoperative period. If the condition will last only until the patient is awake (secretion, etc.), intubation of the patient in the recovery room will often suffice. Other conditions that will last longer should be handled by an orderly tracheotomy. Steroids should be given intraoperatively if the procedure is extensive enough to produce edema. Large resections often also require antibiotic coverage with a broad spectrum antibiotic. (Penicillin or ampicillin in nonallergic patients is usually a good choice.) This will prevent secondary infection and the resultant edema and crusting.

POSTOPERATIVE CONSIDERATIONS

Airway patency during the immediate postoperative period should be carefully and frequently assessed. Recovery room and floor personnel should be aware of signs of upper airway obstruction. If steroids are used, familiarity with their duration of action is necessary as well as airway reassessment should repeat doses become necessary. A portable chest x-ray should be obtained, particularly if the procedure was difficult or extensive resection was performed. Humidity should be used to prevent drying of secretions and crusting. All personnel should be aware of proper suctioning techniques and clear and concise orders should be written for this and for all areas of the airway care. Excessive bleeding should be reported immediately. Reintubation or tracheotomy should be performed if the patient's airway is in jeopardy.

GENERAL MEDICAL CARE

Fluid and electrolyte balance must be properly maintained to prevent dehydration or congestive heart failure. Ongoing preoperative medication must be assessed and reinstituted as indicated.

SPECIFIC COMPLICATIONS—DIAGNOSIS AND TREATMENT

While not intended to be a complete list or a thorough discussion of diagnosis and treatment, the following complications occur with enough frequency to warrant a brief discussion of diagnosis and treatment.

Laryngospasm/Bronchospasm.—These are usually secondary to irritation of the tracheobronchial tree. Often spasm will occur during recovery from anesthesia in the operating room, but may occur later if secretions or blood irritate the tracheobronchial tree. Patients with known asthma are particularly susceptible. The diagnosis of laryngospasm is suspected when laryngeal stridor is present on inspiration. Examination reveals the cords in apposition. Initially, mask ventilation may be difficult or impossible. A to-and-fro wheezing is audible on auscultation when bronchospasm occurs. Mask ventilation is similarly difficult. The condition may be prevented by the use of topical anesthesia (4% cocaine) in a spray. In asthmatics, bronchodilating agents used in the preoperative period are helpful. Most cases of laryngospasm or bronchospasm resolve spontaneously. Those that do not respond in a reasonable length of time to mask pressure may require neuromuscular blocking agents with reintubation or bronchodilators.

Injury to Teeth, Gums, Tongue, Dentures.—Careful inspection after endoscopy will reveal most of these. Hairline fractures of the teeth may not become apparent for a considerable time after the procedure. Dental consultation should be obtained as soon as possible. Dislodged teeth should be recovered and saved. All denture restorations should be checked carefully. Destroyed teeth should be recovered with further endoscopy if necessary.

Lacerations to the tongue or gingivae usually heal spontaneously. If the laceration is large, it should be loosely closed with absorbable suture. Hematomas of tongue may require a nasopharyngeal airway until resolution.

Lacerations of Mucosa.—Most lacerations of the mucosa can be noted at the time of endoscopy. Lacerations through the pyriform sinus or hypopharyngeal mucosa may produce subcutaneous emphysema or abscess. Neck films can sometimes aid in the diagnosis of such perforations. Most superficial lacerations and small pyriform sinus or hypopharyngeal perforations will also heal spontaneously, although coverage with a broad-spectrum antibiotic is recommended. Rarely, an external drainage procedure will be needed to drain an abscess in the parapharyngeal or retropharyngeal space. Subcutaneous emphysema can compromise the airway and may require reintubation of the patient until it resolves.

Pneumothorax and Pneumomediastinum.—These should be suspected when extensive, difficult, or traumatic endoscopy has occurred. Pneumothorax usually results in respiratory difficulty. Breath sounds will be decreased on the affected side and hyperresonant on the opposite side. Mediastinal shift may be apparent. The diagnosis is confirmed by chest film. Small pneumothoraces that are not expanding usually resolve spontaneously and follow-up examination with chest films should suffice. Larger or expanding pneumothoraces may require tube thoracotomy drainage. A thoracic surgeon should be consulted when the pneumothorax is present.

If pneumomediastinum is large and expanding it may cause decreased cardiac output and decreased heart sounds. The diagnosis is confirmed by chest plate. Most pneumomediastinums resolve spontaneously. Occasionally, if they are expanding or if infection ensues, thoracotomy and drainage is necessary.

Laryngeal, Tracheal, Bronchial Edema.—These should be anticipated with difficult endoscopy or extensive resections. Steroids and bronchodilators minimize these complications. The diagnosis is suggested by the slowly progressing signs of stridor and wheezing. Restlessness and tachycardia in the postoperative endoscopy patient should be assumed to be respiratory obstruction until proven otherwise. Sedation in such a patient, particularly with a medication with known respiratory suppression, i.e., morphine, may precipitate respiratory arrest.

If the airway and pulmonary exchange is adequate, this will usually resolve spontaneously. Intravenous steroids will speed the resolution. If edema is severe and the patient does not respond to steroids or bronchodilators, intubation or tracheotomy might be necessary.

Airway Obstruction due to Secretions, Bleeding, or Crusting.— These may produce either slowly progressive or rapid respiratory obstruction. Prevention by proper humidity, suction, and appropriate antibiotics will reduce this complication.

Bleeding should be controlled if accessible. Elevation of the upper body will enhance respiration. Re-endoscopy may be necessary to control some bleeding and provide for suctioning and irrigation of secretions or crust removal. In rare instances, tracheotomy may be warranted.

CONCLUSIONS

As with most complications, attention to detail in the preoperative, postoperative, and intraoperative period is imperative. This includes careful assessment of the patient and the instruments used, and with appropriate diagnostic and treatment methods to correct underlying conditions. Good communication with both the patient and with all members of the health care team cannot be overemphasized.

Despite all this, complications will occur. Early recognition and treatment of these complications will serve to minimize their effect.

BIBLIOGRAPHY

1. Johnson J.T., Myers E.N.: Recent advances in operative laryngoscopy. *Otolaryngol. Clin. North Am.* 17:35–40, 1984.
2. Jako G.J.: Laryngeal endoscopy and microlaryngoscopy, in Paparella M.M., Shumrick D.A. (eds.): *Otolaryngology*. Philadelphia, W.B. Saunders Co., 1980, pp. 2589–2603.

5 Complications of CO_2 Laser Endoscopy

Marvin P. Fried, M.D.

The CO_2 laser has been proven to be an exceptionally effective surgical instrument in the diagnosis and therapy of disorders of the larynx and tracheobronchial tree. It offers precision and the ability to have access to areas unobtainable by other endoscopic techniques. Its use, however, rests on the visualization of the pathology using standard methods. This alone may be a difficult task, fraught with potential problems, as detailed in chapter 4.

GENERAL PRINCIPLES

It must be assumed that the surgeon is facile and knowledgeable in standard endoscopy prior to the use of the laser. Currently, the CO_2 laser is the most effective and commonly used of the laser instruments available for airway surgery. The potentials of the Nd:YAG laser are being explored (see chapter 8), but this laser has not gained widespread use. The properties of the CO_2 laser require that it be used with rigid endoscopes. Fiberoptic cables cannot adequately transmit CO_2 laser energy as yet. This constrains, to some extent, the applications of the CO_2 laser. The appropriately sized endoscope must be used; however, in certain circumstances, there are definite limitations of exposure. This is inherent in esophageal disorders in which the CO_2 laser has not been of great value. This is because of the difficulty in visualizing the extent of the pathology as well as the inability to keep normal tissue out of the path of the laser beam. The esophagus, therefore, being a collapsible, muscular structure does not lend itself to this type of surgery.

Other instrumentation factors must be considered. An appropriate suspension system is mandatory to free the surgeon's hands during laryngoscopy. The Lewy laryngoscope holder is not a true suspension device, using the teeth as a fulcrum rather than suspending the larynx from above. The Killian Gallows system or the Boston University modification of this principle eliminates the torsion on the teeth but may be cumbersome in certain patients.[1] Certain anatomical considerations such as mandible configuration and spinal column flexibility limit the type of laryngoscope that can afford the best visualization. Many modifications have been designed, the best usually incorporating the anterior commissure design, the widest possible body, a build-in suction port, and oxidized metal to prevent laser reflection, as well as excellent illumination cables.

Bronchoscopes for laser use are adaptations of those generally available. The difficulty in maneuverability is compounded during bronchoscopy in which one of the surgeon's hands must support the endoscope, leaving the other to control and aim the laser. Instrumentation down the scope is awkward, especially if the laser plume as well as blood must be evacuated for adequate visualization. Any laser system adds bulk to the proximal end of the bronchoscope, thereby changing the balance of the instrument. Binocular vision is impossible in bronchoscopy and often sacrificed during laryngoscopy at higher magnification. Patient head and neck position may need to be altered frequently during bronchoscopy, requiring knowledgeable assistants available in the operating room.

New endoscopic instruments are constantly being added to the surgical armamentarium to allow for better visualization and control down a relatively narrow tube.[2, 3] The appropriate forceps, suction tips, scissors, spatulas, vocal cord protectors or platforms, and even cautery or microclips must be chosen prior to the procedure. The surgeon cannot leave the setting up and testing of the laser to the nursing staff alone. He or she should be knowledgeable in its use, sources of failure, and the simple "trouble-shooting" measures required. Alternative plans should be available in case the laser fails to function properly.

Even in the best of circumstances, certain areas in the airway are difficult to visualize. These include the subglottis and undersurface of the vocal cords, the laryngeal ventricles, and the posterior commissure, especially with an endotracheal tube in place.[4] Areas not seen cannot be reached with the laser. Therefore, the surgeon must be mindful that many methods are available and assess each case as to the applicability of the use of the laser when compared with the alternatives. The laser should offer at least the same benefit, if not greater advantage, in any particular situation, rather than using it "because it is there."

THE LASER AND SOFT-TISSUE DESTRUCTION

The effect of the laser on the surgical site must be kept in mind when limitations are considered. With the transformation of light energy to thermal energy, tissue temperatures are rapidly increased and evaporation occurs. The potential scatter of cellular debris to surrounding tissue does not seem to occur. Shrinking, curling, and cavity formation are produced with carbonization of solid components and minimal production of apparently nonviable cells.[5] This has direct bearing on the potential of local spread of tumor cells.

The thermal effects on the soft tissue is dependent on the duration of exposure and power of the laser, with larger ulcers and deeper necrosis directly proportional to these parameters.[6,7] The surgeon must therefore constantly observe the character of the tissue being lasered. The deeper the laser incision, the greater the potential for scarring or penetration outside of the airway. This may occur in the larynx as well as the tracheobronchial tree.

One benefit to the use of the laser is the excellent hemostasis it affords. Blood vessels smaller than 0.5 mm in diameter are sealed with similar effects to lymphatic channels.[8] Postoperative edema is reduced; however, larger vessels will not be controlled, causing bleeding at the time of surgery or delayed bleeding. The concomitant use of hemostatic microclips or electrocoagulation is mandatory in these situations.[9] This will reduce the likelihood of delayed hemorrhage, which can be disastrous in the airway.

Last, no matter how delicate the technique or minimal the tissue disruption, healing always produces some scar formation. In tubular structures, such as the subglottis or trachea, this scarring will lead to subsequent cicatrix and stenosis. Circumferential lasering must therefore be avoided.

INDICATIONS FOR LASER ENDOSCOPIC SURGERY

Benign Disease

Recurrent Respiratory Papillomatosis

Recurrent respiratory papillomatosis is most often a disease of childhood, although any age may be affected.

It is the most common benign tumor of the larynx. Papillomas most frequently involve the larynx and tracheobronchial tree, causing hoarseness and varying degrees of respiratory obstruction. Spontaneous remissions are known to occur; however, respiratory papillomatosis is usually progressive, requiring multiple courses of therapy. The etiology remains uncertain, however, a viral association has been postulated. Multiple methods of treatment have been attempted. Medically, these include podophyllin, hormones, chemotherapy (such as 5-fluorouracil) and topical medications.[10] Immunotherapy with the use of vaccines (autogenous, bovine, and bacillus Calmette-Guerin), levamisole, and interferon have been attempted. Of these, interferon seems to be the most promising.[11,12] Cauterization, ultrasound, cryosurgery, and irradiation (no longer used) have been tried with varying success.[10] No curative treatment is available and surgical removal of the papilloma is often necessary to maintain a patent airway. In many patients multiple surgical procedures are necessary. The objective is therefore to preserve as much of the normal structures as possible, thereby preserving normal function, without seeding papilloma into the distal airways, and attempting to avoid a tracheotomy.

The laser is ideally suited for use in this disorder because of the precision it affords, the minimal scarring it produces, and its hemostatic effect.[13] Reduction in tumor burden or viral particles may also play a beneficial role.[12]

Although the potential for spreading papilloma from the larynx to the tracheobronchial trees is a theoretical possibility with Venturi jet ventilation, Simpson and Strong[13] have not found this to be a clinical reality. Lasered particles should be removed no matter what type of anesthetic technique is used. This prevents internal combustion of an endotracheal tube, the obstruction of suction tips, and excessively high (100° C) tissue temperatures. Endoscopy must maintain adequate ventilation working from distal to proximal and avoiding circumferential lasering.

Laryngotracheal Stenosis

Scarring of the larynx and trachea can occur at any level and from a myriad of causes. External trauma, such as a crush injury or internal trauma from prolonged endotracheal intubation are two examples. Partial laryngeal surgery for neoplasm can lead to unexpected fibrosis compromising laryngeal function and narrowing the airway. Initial treatment must control the airway (often by tracheotomy) and address the underlying abnormality (such as realigning a fractured larynx). Infection may require appropriate antibiotic coverage.

Correction of the stenosis can then be managed by open procedures as well as endoscopically. Stenosis severe enough to cause severe respiratory obstruction is difficult to treat by either modality, however, when appropriately used, the laser can avoid an external approach. Potentially, the laser may delay collagen formation by allowing early epithelization. This possible laser benefit is not as important when large stenotic areas are involved.[15]

The benefit of the laser in effectively resecting supraglottic scar has been clearly demonstrated.[16, 17] This may involve epiglottectomy or excision of fibrous bands at the false cord level. Swelling can be minimized using a relatively atraumatic procedure. Indeed, of all of the locations in the airway, supraglottic surgery for stenosis seems most amenable to laser therapy.

Glottic stenosis presents a more difficult problem. Accurate preoperative assessment of the degree of obstruction is imperative. Evaluation of arytenoid mobility must be performed before the therapeutic decisions can be made. Overzealous resection of scar tissue may lead to an incompetent larynx and subsequent aspiration. This is compounded by arytenoid immobility. The use of soft stents (e.g., Silastic®) is required to prevent restenosis. The duration of stenting is uncertain, however, six weeks has proven effective.[18] Steroids and antibiotics seem to minimize tissue reaction to a foreign object and thereby diminish granulation tissue formation.

Subglottic stenosis may be the most difficult management problem. The presence of adequate cartilaginous support must be evaluated. Endoscopic therapy will usually fail if insufficient external architecture is present to stabilize a new lumen.[19] Severe subglottic or tracheal stenosis cannot be managed adequately with the laser alone. In these situations a pedicled hyoid graft interposition into the anterior cricoid and/or tracheal wall has been successful. Stenting is usually required. A tracheotomy may need to be lowered. Both a Montgomery T-tube and rolled Silastic® sheeting have been effective in this situation. A soft-tissue lateral radiograph of the neck taken after six to eight weeks may show air around the T-tube, suggesting an adequate airway allowing stent removal.

Laryngeal stenosis, frequently in the subglottis, often occurs in the pediatric age group. Congenital stenosis due to a cricoid malformation cannot be corrected endoscopically. Stenosis secondary to scarring, however, can be effectively treated with the laser.[18, 20]

Benign Tumors

Precise excision of benign tumors can be accomplished with the laser. The surgeon must be cognizant that many of these lesions can be adequately treated by other modalities. An example would be vocal nodules, which, because of their small size, can be removed by cup forceps as well as the laser.

Polypoid swelling of the vocal cords is a common occurrence, frequently due to voice abuse, noxious stimuli (e.g., cigarette smoke) or other chronic environmental irritants. Often both cords are diffusely involved. If the laser is used for resection, then consideration should be given to staged procedure. Although the surgeon may be able to remove the edematous and redundant tissue from both the vocal cords, the resultant prolonged voice alterations make vocal rehabilitation difficult. In this circumstance, staged procedures, first operating in one cord, and then the other weeks later, may be a prudent decision. Subsequent web formation is also avoided. If the base of the polyp is narrow, sparing the anterior commissure, then bilateral excision may be accomplished at one procedure.

The CO_2 laser is effective in treating subglottic capillary hemangiomas, avoiding tracheotomy. Excessive bleeding may be encountered in the cavenous type when laser excision is performed.[21] Small lesions often respond to a few laser procedures; however, larger tumors (supraglottic and transglottic) may require multiple attempts at removal.[22] There is hardly any other method of resecting these tumors endoscopically that gives the surgeon as much control and accuracy.

Other tumors such as xanthoma (Fig 5–1), neurofibroma (Fig 5–2), and granular cell myoblastoma have been removed, often avoiding an external approach. Granulation tissue may form near the posterior commissure from prolonged intubation or at the internal margins of a tracheotomy (Fig 5–3). Laser removal in these situations is hemostatic and accurate. Marsupialization of internal laryngoceles is easily accomplished and should be performed during quiescence to avoid the later formation of a laryngopyocele.

Other Conditions

Various surgical methods have been suggested for prevention of aspiration.[23] Few of these can be reversed to allow for return of voice and removal of a tracheotomy tube. The epiglottic flap technique can be partially

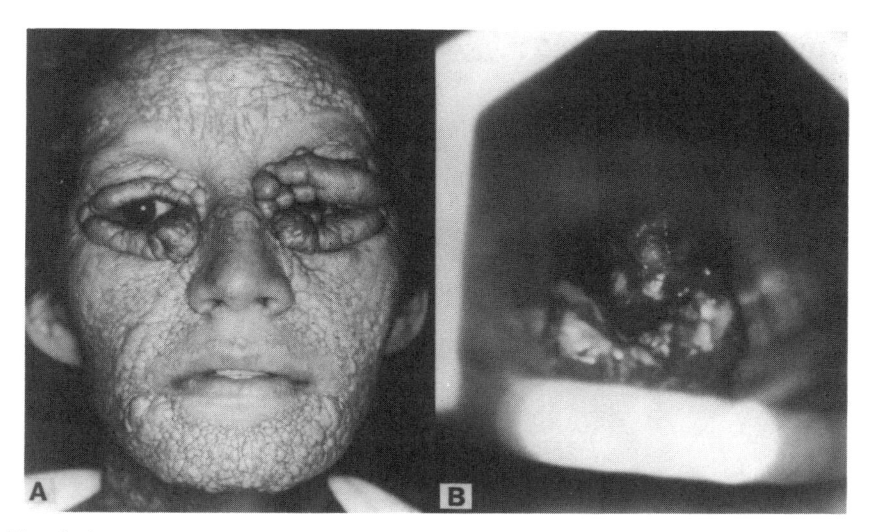

Fig 5–1. Patient with diffuse xanthomatosis **(A)** and laryngeal endoscopic appearance **(B).**

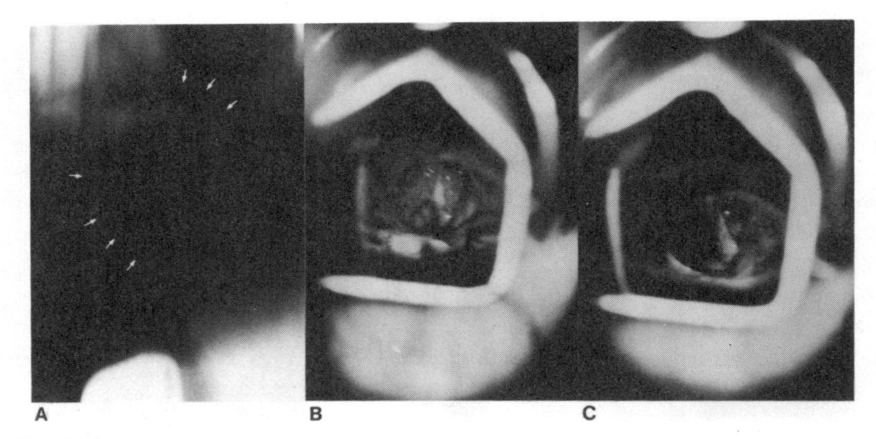

Fig 5–2. Lateral polytomograph of 17-year-old male patient with neurofibromatosis showing supraglottic lesion **(A).** Endoscopic views of supraglottic neurofibroma obstructing the laryngeal inlet, before **(B),** and after **(C)** laser debulking.

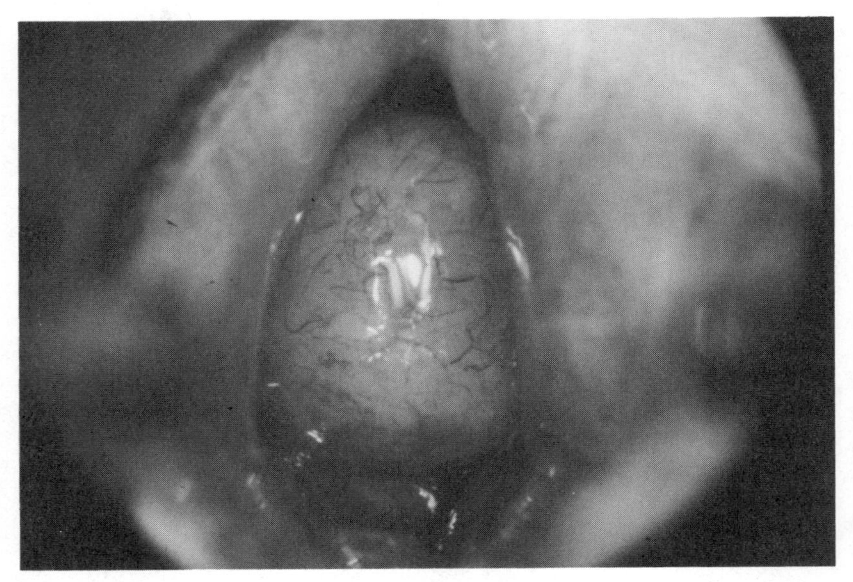

Fig 5–3. Polypoid granulation tissue appearing in the subglottis in a patient with a tracheotomy.

or totally reversed by resection or a portion of all of the epiglottis. We have found this can be achieved with the laser, other methods being unsatisfactory (Fig 5–4).

Endoscopic laser arytenoidectomy can be performed for bilateral vocal cord paralysis.[24,25] In this situation, the degree of resection can be well controlled; however, due to the inherent limitations of the optical system, the surgical procedure is often longer than anticipated. This is because of the difficulty in maneuvering the arytenoid into alignment with the beam. Moreover, the muscular attachments to the arytenoid are numerous, requiring frequent changes in position. Nonetheless, resection of the arytenoid can be accomplished with airway improvement. Care must be taken not to expose the posterior commissure so that webbing, which limits the beneficial result, does not occur.

Epiglottectomy for benign lesions is an effective technique. This has been described for patients with perichondritis and persistent supraglottic

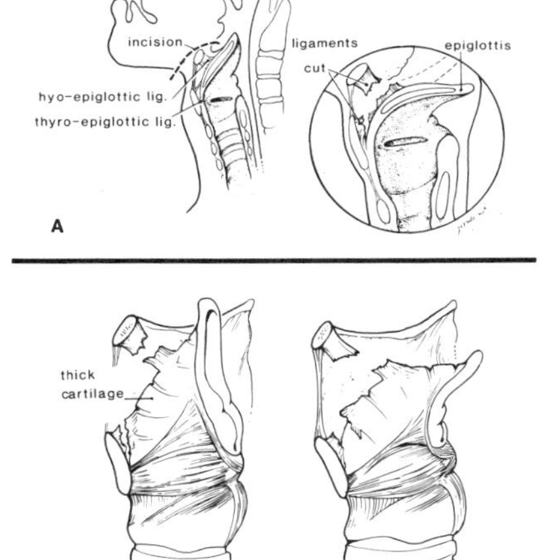

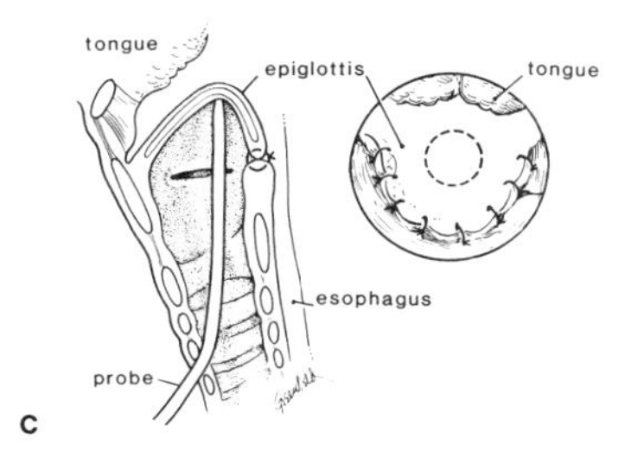

Fig 5–4. The creation of the epiglottic flap necessitates cutting the hypoepiglottic and thyroepiglottic ligaments *(a* and *b).* Reversal of this technique is possible with the laser. Tenting epiglottis from below affords view of area to be opened *(c).* (From Strome M., Fried M.P.: Rehabilitative surgery for aspiration: A clinical analysis. *Arch. Otolaryngol.* 109:809–811, 1983. Used by permission.)

edema for disorders such as Crohn's disease. Airway improvement occurs rapidly with the potential for decannulation of tracheotomy-dependent patients.[26]

Another possible use of the laser is creation of a tracheoesophageal fistula for a voice prosthesis after total laryngectomy. At this time, however, control of fistula placement seems to be more accurate with the puncture technique.[27, 28]

Premalignant and Malignant Disease

Diagnosis

As experience has increased with endoscopic laser surgery for benign disease, the capabilities of this instrument in both premalignant and malignant disorders has also undergone evolution. Although the laryngologist can be suspicious that any particular lesion that exhibits leukoplakia or erythroplasia may be less than a frank malignancy, certainty lies only in biopsy. Both cigarette smoking and alcohol consumption are strong cofactors in the mucosal metamorphosis to laryngeal and hypopharyngeal carcinoma.[29] The findings of a suspicious lesion in a 60-year-old man with an exposure history as just noted certainly requires biopsy diagnosis. This situation may be typical, but neoplasia may occur in either sex, at most any age without a history of smoking or alcohol consumption. At the other end of the spectrum is the patient with diffuse mucosal disease, many areas being potentially malignant. A biopsy is indicated in all of these circumstances.

Diagnostically, tissue samples are easily obtained using the laser with the added benefit of hemostasis. The tissue remaining *in situ* can undergo minimal manipulation thereby, theoretically at least, diminishing the possibility of tumor spread. As the biopsy specimens are taken, margins can be assessed.[30] Anterior commissure involvement can be traced into cartilage, altering staging from T1 to T4.[31] This assessment of the depth of penetration can be suggested by the characteristics of the tissue as it is being lasered, as muscle gives way to the "sparkle" of cartilage. Bulky, exophytic tumors can be vaporized to assist in the delineation of mucosal extension. Partial excision can similarly be accomplished avoiding an initial tracheotomy when the airway is compromised before therapy is begun. This has the benefit of eliminating the potential for stomal seeding of tumor or the infection that may result.[32] It also prevents more thoughtful therapeutic planning, since no "bridges are burned." It must be remembered that the avoidance of a tracheotomy should not jeopardize the patency of the airway. This must be secure even in the presence of partially obstructing lesions. Laser surgery does not take the place of tracheotomy in severe respiratory distress.

Therapy

Premalignant mucosal alteration can be diffuse. The laser allows for judicious sampling and resection without overtreatment. Because of the minimal tissue reaction, biopsy specimens can be obtained in multiple sites so that a true malignancy is not overlooked.

The anatomic limitations of laser cordectomy have been defined by Davis and co-workers.[31] The most important factor is the thyroid cartilage, which allows but 2 to 3 mm of soft tissue at the anterior commissure. Increasing tissue depth is obtained with more posterior extension, the thyroid ala again acting as the lateral boundary. The cricothyroid membrane is the inferior limit and the para-arytenoid musculature the posterolateral demarcation. Within those anatomic limits, vocal cord function and laryngeal competency can be preserved. Excessive removal of the thyroarytenoid muscle, ventricular folds, or epiglottis can lead to continuous aspiration compounded if arytenoid cartilage is excised.

Laser surgery of glottic laryngeal carcinoma (T1 tumors) is not appropriate for all patients. Certain beneficial criteria should be met if curative therapy is sought with only laser excision, as suggested by Vaughan[30]: the tumor must be completely visualized by laryngoscopy; the vocal cord or vocal process of the arytenoid should be free of tumor; the lesion should be confined to the mucous membrane; high magnification should disclose no further disease after excision; frozen-section specimens are free of tumor after excision; and margins are free after permanent section.

Phonotory function and quality following laser cordectomy is quite satisfactory. Normalcy is not obtained. However, the formation of a pseudocord achieves vocal characteristics within the normal male register.[33]

The curative results of laser cordectomy for T1 tumors has been encouraging, with 92% three-year control in selected patients.[30] This excellent result requires careful staging and complete familiarity with the capabilities and limitations of the laser. Other therapeutic modalities such as radiation therapy can yield similar results with minimal morbidity.[34] The efficiency, patient cost, and potential alteration of surrounding otherwise normal tissue must be considered when comparing surgery with radiation.

Small supraglottic (epiglottic) lesions may be excised, however, the potential for lymphatic spread for these lesions, especially those involving the aryepiglottic fold, when compared with glottic malignancy, is much greater. The possibility of nodal disease must not be overlooked in the attempts at controlling the primary tumor. Lesions extending to the infrahyoid epiglottis may involve the pre-epiglottic space and should not be treated by epiglottectomy alone.[35]

Newer concepts of multimodality therapy have also involved the laser.

Advanced or recurrent carcinomas of the upper airway have been treated with combined laser surgery and radiation therapy. The rapid healing subsequent to laser procedures permits early institution of radiation with marked cytoreduction, even if just for palliation. Feldman and associates[36] have reported good to excellent local tolerance of combined therapy in seven of ten patients (six of the ten having laryngeal tumors). Even though T3 tumors cannot be treated solely with the laser, the possibility of combined therapy may be realistic in certain situations. It is judicious to allow the effects of radiation to subside prior to any subsequent endoscopic surgery. Tissue planes are more clearly defined and edema is reduced. If the thyroid cartilage must be sacrificed, then an external partial laryngectomy (hemilaryngectomy or subtotal supragottic laryngectomy) needs to be performed. This can be done for recurrent tumor, even after an endoscopic procedure.

CO_2 LASER BRONCHOSCOPY

Various laser systems have been used to treat tumors of the tracheobronchial tree. The newest is the argon rhodamine-B dye laser used in conjunction with a hematoporphyrin derivative to photoradiate endobronchial tumors.[37] The hematoporphyrin that has been previously administered is concentrated in the tumor. The tissue is acted on by the laser delivered by a fiber threaded down a bronchoscope and which results in specific photosensitivity and destruction. This method lacks depth of tissue penetration, and tumor cell death does not go beyond 2 cm. The possibilities of greater specificity and tissue ablation are based on refined hematoporphyrins that are being developed.[38] This method holds great promise for various sites in the head and neck as well because of specificity and accessibility.

The Nd:YAG laser for bronchoscopy is dealt with in great detail by in chapter 8.

The CO_2 laser has been attached to a rigid bronchoscope since 1973[39] (Fig 5–5). Its greatest usefulness has been in the treatment of respiratory papillomatosis of the trachea and bronchi.[40] The hemostasis achieved, with minimal tumor handling and edema, are as advantageous in the thorax as they are in the larynx. Multiple procedures are often required, often to maintain a patent airway.

Benign lesions can be excised, often avoiding a more extensive open resection. An example is depicted in Figure 5–6 of a 32-year-old woman with symptoms of chronic obstructive pulmonary disease, who in reality had a granular cell tumor of the trachea, removed by laser surgery in two operations. Tracheal stenosis is a more difficult problem. Rarely are single

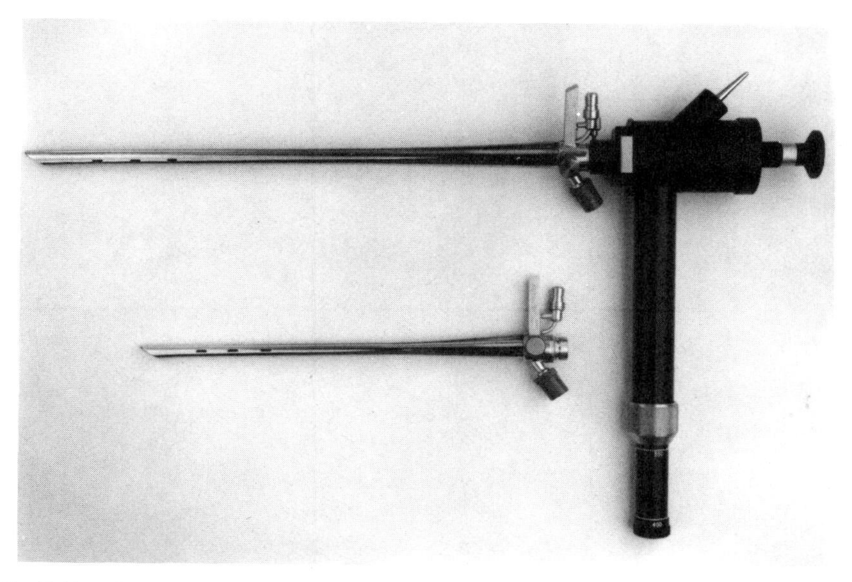

Fig 5–5. One available model of the laser bronchoscope. (From Thaller S., Fried M.P., Goodman M.L.: *Chest* 88:925–928, 1985. Used by permission.

attempts therapeutic. Dilatation often must accompany endoscopic laser resection along with placement of a stent whether of T-tube variety or rolled Silastic.®

Obstructing malignant tumors of the trachea and bronchi are amenable to laser resection, whether by the CO_2 or Nd:YAG laser. The clinical circumstance must be appropriate: a resectable primary tumor that can be reduced by initial intraluminal excision or a nonresectable lesion that is producing airway obstruction and laser surgery offers palliation.[38] The diagnosis can be achieved with the laser owing to the hemostatic effect. Various tumors have been treated, whether primary in the lung, such as squamous cell or small cell carcinoma, adenocarcinoma or adenocystic carcinoma,[40,41] or metastatic disease such as melanoma.[42] In order for the laser to be effective, the tumor must be endoluminal and not solely compressing the airway externally and accessible by rigid bronchoscopy. Therefore distal bronchi and upper lobe segments are difficult, if not impossible, to treat currently. The Nd:YAG laser can reach these areas, and the future may hold a CO_2 laser delivered through a fiberoptic cable.

Laser resection of these malignancies is not curative nor meant to be. Immediate benefit is obtained in many patients with impaired airway patency as well as reversal of atelectatic pulmonary parenchyma obstructed by endobronchial disease. Laser "unblocking" of the airway can lead to effec-

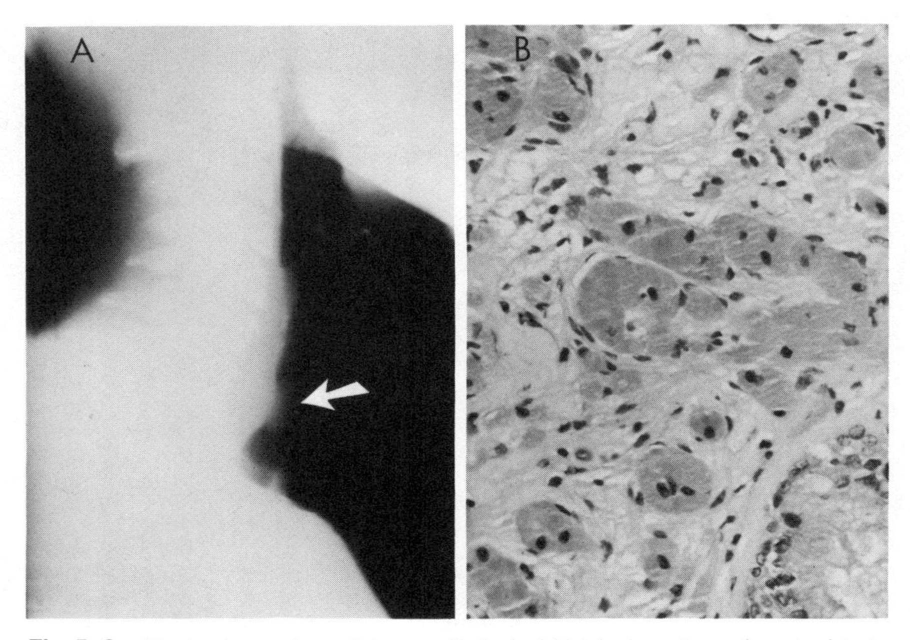

Fig 5–6. Tracheal granular cell tumor with typical histologic pattern. *Arrow* points to man with almost tracheal obstruction *(a)*.

tive radiation therapy by eliminating dyspnea and pneumonitis.[40] Difficulties arise in those patients who are often quite ill. Massive hemorrhage may be difficult to control. Postoperative edema or the release of secretions may overwhelm an already compromised airway. The manipulation of a rigid bronchoscope with the attached laser may be difficult in some patients, and the need for suction to remove blood and vapor and the precise alignment of the laser beam may be cumbersome to accomplish. These technical problems will probably be overcome with advances in instrument design, both within the bronchoscope and with laser coupling.

COMPLICATIONS OF CO_2 LASER ENDOSCOPY

As the laser gains more frequent utility, the incidence of actual as well as theoretical complications will increase. Numerous difficulties involving laser procedures have already been reported. The most catastrophic have involved endotracheal tube fires. Individual experiences of complications may not adequately reflect the general consensus. Healy and his associates[43] have been performing laser surgery since 1971 and have recently reported nine complications in a total of 4,416 cases, representing a complication rate of 0.2%. Six of these problems related to fires, one facial burn due to an overheated bronchoscope, and two due to hemorrhage.

Another retrospective analysis has been performed by Ossoff and his colleagues[44] at Northwestern University Medical School. Of 204 cases involving all types of CO_2 laser surgery, 12 complications arose. Two complications were sustained by OR staff (finger burns). Six laser-related patient problems occurred involving retained metallic tape in the oropharynx, perichondritis with posterior web formation, and laser burn of a tooth, and two cases of postoperative airway obstruction occurred (one due to edema and one due to a retained pharyngeal pack). The remaining complications were related to laryngeal suspension causing edema, tooth trauma, or facial pressure sores. None of these untoward events were life-threatening; however, the surgeons were meticulous in their laser technique.

A broader experience has been reported by Fried.[45] The members of one of the senior otolaryngology societies were surveyed by mail. Of 229 questionnaires mailed, 210 (92%) were returned. Of these physicians, 27% did not use the laser and an additional 49% used the laser without complications. Most of these otolaryngologists used the laser less than six times per month. The remaining 49 physicians (27%) reported a total of 81 complications (Table 5–1) including endotracheal explosion, laryngeal stenosis

TABLE 5–1.—CO_2 LASER COMPLICATIONS[45]

COMPLICATION	NO.
Endotracheal explosion	28
Laryngeal web	15
Facial burn	9
Pneumothorax	5
Laryngeal stenosis	4
Endotracheal cuff ignition	3
Postoperative hemorrhage	3
Subglottic stenosis	3
Cottonoid ignition	2
Subcutaneous emphysema	2
Laryngeal edema	2
Tracheal stenosis	1
Endobronchial explosion	1
Perichondritis	1
Carbon granuloma	1
Pharyngeal burn	1
Total	**81**

or web formation, facial burns, and hemorrhage. Five cases of pneumothorax and two of subcutaneous emphysema were also reported. Surprisingly, increased experience with the laser did not necessarily guarantee fewer complications. On the basis of this survey, it is apparent that the few reports of complications of laser laryngoscopy does not reflect the true incidence of untoward events. It is also apparent that the surgical dictum of increased experience leading to fewer complications does not hold true for this type of procedure. The general number of complications reflected the number of cases performed per month.

The spectrum of complications can be conceptualized into direct, secondary, and delayed effects (Table 5–2). The most frequent, and perhaps the most serious of the direct effects, is the ignition of the endotracheal tube and the consequent effects.[45–52] This can occur with direct impact on the outside of an unprotected tube or in a dehiscence in the wrapping. Another method of ignition is by the insufflation of tissue embers into the lumen of the tube causing internal combustion in an obviously unprotected surface, a secondary effect. The severity of this injury depends not only on the duration and extent of the burn within the patient, but also the composition of the endotracheal tubes. Although various studies have shown benefits of one tube

TABLE 5–2.—CO_2 LASER COMPLICATIONS[45]

Direct Laser Effects
Burn of tissue out of operative field (e.g., eye, facial)
Mucosal burn
Endotracheal tube ignition
Ignition of cottonoid
Pneumothorax
Subcutaneous emphysema
Second Laser Effects
Endotracheal tube obstruction by lasered tissue
Endotracheal tube ignition by flaming tissue
Burn from a reflecting surface
Outside of laryngoscope
Within laryngoscope
Mucosal charring with airway obstruction
Hemorrhage
Edema
Perichondritis
Delayed Laser Effects
Vocal cord web
Cicatrix and stenosis (laryngeal, tracheal)
Glottic incompetence due to excessive tissue removal

over another, the polyvinylchloride (PVC) tube produces more severe injury than other materials. Ignition is more rapid with PVC tubes when compared with red rubber tubes[52] and soft-tissue effects are more destructive.[53] Moreover, hydrochloride gas is a product of PVC combustion and as a respiratory irritant can lead to distal pulmonary parenchymal damage.[45,51]

Other direct effects include burns to the eye, face, or mucosa, as well as ignition of other substances in the operative field, such as cottonoids placed in the airway. Perforation of the tracheal wall may occur as a consequence of tissue erosion by the pathological process being treated, or by the continuous use of the laser itself. In another chapter, Healy depicts such a case with another having already been reported in detail[54] or tabulated on the survey discussed above.[45] The use of a Venturi system when a tracheal perforation does occur, can lead to massive subcutaneous emphysema, as well as bilateral pneumothoraces.

Secondary laser effects occur as a result of tissue alteration produced by the laser or laser instrumentation. The endotracheal tube can become obstructed, either by mucus or by lasered tissue.[55] Tissue can be burned by the laser light reflected off the endoscope, either outside or within the lumen. Other secondary effects include edema, perichondritis, and granuloma formation.[56] The aluminum wrapping surrounding the endotracheal tube may loosen and then dislodge in the distal airway, causing obstruction.[57] If the wrap is not meticulous, not only will the underlying tube be exposed, but the rough metallic tape edges can cause damage to the nasal mucosa in nasotracheal intubation, with subsequent epistaxis, and also lacerations to the pharynx and larynx.[58]

Burns to the oral cavity and lips may occur when the entire endotracheal (E-T) tube ignites. Facial burns also may develop when the bronchoscope that is resting on the patient's cheek becomes heated by the laser.

Delayed problems involve cordal webs produced when the anterior commissure and both vocal cords are lasered. If a subglottic stenosis is excised and circumferential mucosa is denuded, a cicatrix may form, causing even further stenosis. Excessive tissue removal for vocal cord carcinoma or for arytenoidectomy may leave the glottis incompetent with subsequent aspiration.[59]

If a complication should arise, assessment of the extent of injury should be made as soon as possible. If an airway fire occurs, the source of oxygen should be disconnected immediately and the endotracheal tube should be removed. Ventilation should be continued with a smaller cuffed tube. Laryngoscopy and bronchoscopy should then be performed to remove any debris and evaluate the injury. If there are extensive mucosal burns, antibiotics and steroids are of value. Ventilatory support may be necessary. Continued care depends on the individual situation and the extent of the injury. In severe cases, reverse isolation, tracheal cultures, repeated endoscopy, and intensive support may be required. Pulmonary parenchymal damage may need to be evaluated with appropriate radiographs (polytomography, CT scanning), blood gas determinations, and ventilation profusion scans.[46]

Although the laser surgical team must be aware of measures to be taken in case of a laser problem, emphasis must be placed on prevention. Preparation (Table 5–3) should include preoperative team discussion as well as familiarity with the equipment to be used. The operation of the laser must be checked before it is used on the patient with the spot size, CO_2 laser, and aiming beam aligned at the outset. Alternative surgical techniques should be considered as well as the steps to be taken should a fire occur. Eye protection should be afforded to the patient (moist eye pads) as well as the OR personnel (plexiglass or glass eyewear) (Table 5–4). Steroids (dexamethasone 4 to 10 mg, IV) have been useful when administered early in the procedure in preventing laryngeal edema.

Anesthesia precautions (Table 5–5) include a carefully wrapped red rubber E-T tube, smooth and without dehiscences. Polyvinylchloride tubes should be avoided and Venturi ventilation used whenever possible. Water or saline should be placed within the E-T tube cuff as a heat sink and extinguisher.[60] The E-T tube should be kept away from the site of lasering. This may be difficult to manage in the posterior commissure. Any area of the tube not protected by aluminum wrapping tube should be covered with moist cottonoids, kept wet during the procedure. Indeed, everything that is possibly combustible should be kept moist.

TABLE 5–3.—PREVENTION OF COMPLICATIONS—PREPARATION

Discuss care with team members
Become familiar with equipment
Select alternative methods in case of failure
Plan strategy in case of complication (e.g., ignition)
Align aiming beam at outset of each case
Use steroids to decrease edema
Use OR staff eye protection

TABLE 5–4.—PREVENTION OF COMPLICATIONS—PATIENT PREPARATION

Eye protection
Moisten combustibles
Have patient's face covered with moist gauze or cloth
Appropriate position on OR table
Cardiac monitoring for possible prolonged endoscopy

TABLE 5–5.—PREVENTION OF COMPLICATIONS—ANESTHESIA

Carefully wrap E-T tube—smooth without dehiscences
Avoid polyvinylchloride tube
Use water in E-T tube cuff
Venturi ventilation
Keep E-T tube away from site of lasering
Cover E-T cuff with moist cottonoids

TABLE 5–6.—PREVENTION OF COMPLICATIONS—TECHNIQUE

Use binocular vision whenever possible
Keep laser in center of operative field
Begin lasering at low power and brief duration
Reposition laser and laryngoscope as necessary
Observe character of tissue lasered
Remove lasered tissue
Control hemorrhage
Cord protection to prevent webs
Avoid 360° lasering
Remove steam as frequently as needed

Not only should the patient's eyes be covered, but the remaining face as well, in order to prevent stray facial burns by the laser or an overheated endoscope. Suspension of the laryngoscope must be satisfactory for visualization at the outset, with the patient appropriately positioned on the operating table (see chapter 4). Since the vagal response of prolonged laryngeal stimulation may cause a cardiac arrhythmia or even silent ischemia, cardiac monitoring is imperative.[61]

The surgeon must use binocular vision whenever possible (Table 5–6). If repositioning of the patient or the instrumentation is necessary for adequate visualization, it must be accomplished before further lasering is performed. Although laser power at the tissue level depends on exposure time as well as power output, it is most advisable to use the highest possible power with the shortest exposure time to minimize charring and heat transfer to surrounding tissue.[62] Before this is achieved it is advisable to begin lasering at low power and brief duration, working up to a higher power as the surgeon becomes more familiar with the individual patient's tissue response. Overheating of tissue can also be avoided by not repeatedly working in the same operative site, but rather skipping to various sites in the field.

The surgeon should be mindful of tissue response and observe the characteristics of tissue being lasered. Neoplasm behaves differently than mucosa, muscle, or cartilage. This can be used to advantage as experience is gained. It helps to prevent excessive tissue removal, but also can be a clue to deep tumor invasion noted above. Lasered tissue and char should be removed as soon as possible to prevent aspiration into the E-T tube. Char can also be heated to far above 100° C because it is not evaporated by the laser beam.[62] Hemorrhage should be controlled by the use of low laser power, electrocautery, or microclips as bleeding occurs.

The vocal cord not operated on should be protected by appropriate instrumentation so that webs can be prevented. The entire circumference of the subglottis or trachea should not be lasered so that a stenosis is not produced. Excessive tissue should not be removed.[59] Suction should be used to remove vapor as it is produced both to improve vision as well as to prevent reduction of the laser power before it impacts on the tissue.[63] New devices have been developed to give laryngeal suction and protection simultaneously. The use of suction can be accomplished by a side channel in some laryngoscopes.

All of the above precautions and suggestions are designed simply as aids to the endoscopist and laser team. The laser is but an additional surgical tool, as precise as it is. Although complications can and do occur, they are more often attributable to the surgeon rather than the instrument. It is imperative that the physician is properly trained before the laser is used in a clinical setting. This training is offered at many institutions and by highly qualified instructors. Laser safety codes are often established on an individual hospital basis once a unit is purchased.[64] The Laser Safety Committee of the American Academy of Otolaryngology–Head and Neck Surgery is also attempting to formulate recommendations for laser safety standards that can serve as guidelines for individuals and institutions. Complications can be kept to a minimum if the surgeon is well trained, the anesthesiologist aware of the unique nature of laser endoscopy, and the team knowledgeable, with all personnel adhering to detail.

REFERENCES

1. Grundfast K.M., Vaughan C.W., Strong M.S., et al.: Suspension microlaryngoscopy on the Boyce position with a new suspension gallows. *Ann. Otolaryngol. Rhinol. Laryngol.* 87:560–566, 1978.
2. Ossoff R.H., Karlan M.S.: A set of bronchoscopes for carbon dioxide laser surgery. *Otolaryngol. Head Neck Surg.* 91:336–337, 1983.
3. Ossoff R.H., Karlan M.S.: Instrumentation for microlaryngeal laser surgery. *Otolaryngol. Head Neck Surg.* 91:456–460, 1983.

4. Fried M.P.: Limitations of laser laryngoscopy. *Otolaryngol. Clin. North Am.* 17:199–207, 1983.
5. Mihashi S., Hiruno M., Jako G.J., et al.: Interaction of CO_2 laser and soft tissue—the basic mechanism of the carbon dioxide laser irradiation of the soft tissue. *Kurume Med. J.* 27:157–165, 1980.
6. Meyers A.D., Kuzela D.C.: Dose response characteristics of the human larynx with carbon dioxide laser radiation. *Am. J. Otolaryngol.* 1:136–140, 1980.
7. Mihashi S., Jako G.J., Incze J., et al.: Laser surgery in otolaryngology: Interaction of the CO_2 laser in soft tissue. *Ann. N.Y. Acad. Sci.* 267:263–293, 1976.
8. Gillis T.M., Strong M.S.: Surgical lasers and soft tissue interaction. *Otolaryngol. Clin. North Am.* 16:775–784, 1983.
9. Vaughan C.W.: Transoral laryngeal surgery using the CO_2 laser: Laboratory experiments and clinical experience. *Laryngoscope* 88:1399–1920, 1978.
10. Robbins K.T., Woodson G.E.: Current concepts in the management of laryngeal papillomatosis. *Head Neck Surg.* 6:861–866, 1984.
11. Goepfort H., Gutterman J.V., Dichtel W.J., et al.: Leukocyte interferon in patients with juvenile laryngeal papillomatosis. *Ann. Otol. Rhinol. Laryngol.* 91:431–436, 1982.
12. McCabe B.F., Clark K.F.: Interferon and laryngeal papillomatosis: the Iowa experience. *Ann. Otol. Rhinol. Laryngol.* 92:2–7, 1983.
13. Simpson G.T., Strong M.S.: Recurrent respiratory papillomatosis: The role of the carbon dioxide laser. *Otolaryngol. Clin. North Am.* 16:887–894, 1983.
14. Strong M.S., Vaughan C.W., Cooperband S.R., et al.: Recurrent respiratory papillomatosis—management with the CO_2 laser. *Ann. Otol. Rhinol. Laryngol.* 85:508–516, 1976.
15. McGee K.C., Nagle J.W., Toohill R.J.: CO_2 laser repair of subglottic and upper tracheal stenosis. *Otolaryngol. Head Neck Surg.* 89:92–95, 1981.
16. Strong M.S., Healy G.B., Vaughan C.W., et al.: Management of laryngeal stenosis. *Otolaryngol. Clin. North Am.* 12:797–805, 1979.
17. Shugar J.M.A., Som P.M., Biller H.F.: An evaluation of the carbon dioxide laser in the treatment of traumatic laryngeal stenosis. *Laryngoscope* 92:23–26, 1982.
18. Healy G.B.: An experimental model for the endoscopic correction of subglottic stenosis with clinical applications. *Laryngoscope* 92:1103–1115, 1982.
19. Simpson G.T., Strong M.S., Healy G.B., et al.: Predictive factors of success or failure in the endoscopic management of laryngeal and tracheal stenosis. *Ann. Otol. Rhinol. Laryngol.* 91:384–388, 1982.
20. Holinger L.D.: Treatment of severe subglottic stenosis without tracheotomy: A preliminary report. *Ann. Otol. Rhinol. Laryngol.* 91:407–412, 1982.
21. Healy G.B., Fearon B., French R., et al.: Treatment of subglottic hemangioma with the carbon dioxide laser. *Laryngoscope* 90:809–813, 1980.
22. Komisar A., Rubin R.J.: Use of carbon dioxide laser in pediatric otolaryngologic disease. *N.Y. State J. Med.* 81:1761–1764, 1981.
23. Strome M., Fried M.P.: Rehabilitative surgery for aspiration: A clinical analysis. *Arch. Otolaryngol.* 109:809–811, 1983.
24. Eskew J.R., Bailey B.J.: Laser arytenoidectomy for bilateral vocal cord paralysis. *Otolaryngol. Head Neck Surg.* 91:294–298, 1983.

25. Ossoff R.H., Karlan M.S., Sisson G.A.: Endoscopic laser arytenoidectomy. *Lasers Surg. Med.* 2:293–299, 1983.
26. Davis R.K., Shapshay S.M., Strong M.S., et al.: Transoral partial supraglottic resection using the CO_2 laser. *Laryngoscope* 93:429–432, 1983.
27. Singer M.I., Blom E.D.: An endoscopic technique for restoration of voice after laryngectomy. *Ann. Otol. Rhinol. Laryngol.* 89:529–533, 1980.
28. Panje W.R.: Prosthetic vocal rehabilitation following laryngectomy: The voice button. *Ann. Otol. Rhinol. Laryngol.* 90:116–120, 1981.
29. Rothman K.H., Cann C.I., Flanders D., et al.: Epidemiology of laryngeal cancer. *Epidemiol. Rev.* 2:195–209, 1980.
30. Vaughan C.W.: Use of the carbon dioxide laser in the endoscopic management of organic laryngeal disease. *Otolaryngol. Clin. North Am.* 16:849–864, 1983.
31. Davis R.K., Jako G.J., Hyams V.J., et al.: The anatomic limitation of CO_2 laser conducting. *Laryngoscope* 92:980–984, 1982.
32. Davis R.K., Shapshay S.M., Vaughan C.W., et al.: Pretreatment airway management in obstructing carcinoma of the larynx. *Otolaryngol. Head Neck Surg.* 89:209–214, 1981.
33. Vecerina S., Krajina Z.: Phonatory function following unilateral laser cordectomy. *J. Laryngol. Otol.* 97:1139–1144, 1983.
34. Young J.R.: Laser surgery for T1 glottic carcinoma—the argument against. *J. Laryngol. Otol.* 97:243–246, 1983.
35. Nadol J.B. Jr.: Treatment of carcinoma of the epiglottis. *Ann. Otol. Rhinol. Laryngol.* 90:422–448, 1981.
36. Feldman M., Ucmakli A., Strong M.S., et al.: Applications of carbon dioxide laser surgery and radiation. *Arch. Otolaryngol.* 109:240–242, 1983.
37. Hayata Y., Kato H., Konaka C., et al.: Hematoporphyrin derivative and laser photoradiation in the treatment of lung cancer. *Chest* 81:269–277, 1982.
38. Vincent R.G.: Laser therapy for advanced carcinoma of the trachea and bronchus. *Chest* 84:509–510, 1983.
39. Strong M.S., Vaughan C.W., Polangs T., et al.: Bronchoscopic carbon dioxide laser surgery. *Ann. Otol. Rhinol. Laryngol.* 83:769–776, 1974.
40. Shapshay S.M., Simpson G.T.: Lasers in bronchology. *Otolaryngol. Clin. North Am.* 26:879–886, 1983.
41. McElvein R.B., Zorn G.: Treatment of malignant disease in trachea and mainstem bronchi by carbon dioxide laser. *J. Thorac. Cardiovasc. Surg.* 86:858–863, 1983.
42. Andrews A.H. Jr., Caldarelli D.D.: Carbon dioxide laser treatment of metastatic melanoma of the trachea and bronchi. *Ann. Otol. Rhinol. Laryngol.* 90:310–311, 1981.
43. Healy G.B., Strong M.S., Shapshay S., et al.: Complications of CO_2 laser surgery of the aerodigestive tract: Experience of 4416 cases. *Otolaryngol. Head Neck Surg.* 92:13–18, 1984.
44. Ossoff R.H., Hotaling A.J., Karlan M.S., et al.: CO_2 laser in otolaryngology–head and neck surgery: A retrospective analysis of complications. *Laryngoscope* 93:1287–1289, 1983.

45. Fried M.P.: A survey of the complications of laser laryngoscopy. *Arch. Otolaryngol.* 110:31–34, 1984.
46. Schramm V.L. Jr., Mattox D.E., Stool S.E.: Acute management of laser-ignited intratracheal explosion. *Laryngoscope* 91:1417–1426, 1981.
47. Snow J.C., Norton M.L., Saluja T.S., et al.: Fire hazard during CO_2 laser microsurgery on the larynx and trachea. *Anesth. Analg.* 55:146–147, 1976.
48. Vourc'h G., Tannieres M., Freche G.: Ignition of a tracheal tube during laryngeal laser surgery. *Anesthesia* 34:685, 1979.
49. Hirshman C.A., Leon D.: Ignition of an endotracheal tube during laser microsurgery. *Anesthesiology* 53:177, 1980.
50. Hirshman C.A., Smith J.: Indirect ignition of the endotracheal tube during carbon dioxide laser surgery. *Arch. Otolaryngol.* 106:639–641, 1980.
51. Cozine K., Rosenbaum L.M., Askanazi J., et al.: Laser-induced endotracheal tube fire. *Anesthesiology* 55:583–585, 1981.
52. Myers A.: Complication of CO_2 laser surgery of the larynx. *Ann. Otol. Rhinol. Laryngol.* 90:132–134, 1981.
53. Ossoff R.H., Duncavage J.A., Eisenman T.S., et al.: Comparison of tracheal damage from laser-ignited endotracheal tube fires. *Ann. Otol. Rhinol. Laryngol.* 92:333–335, 1983.
54. Ganfield R.A., Chapin J.W.: Pneumothorax with upper airway laser surgery. *Anesthesiology* 56:398–399, 1982.
55. Torres L.E., Reynolds R.C.: A complication of use of a microlaryngeal surgery endotracheal tube. *Anesthesiology* 53:355, 1980.
56. Feder R.J.: Laryngeal granuloma as a complication of the CO_2 laser. *Laryngoscope* 93:944–945, 1983.
57. Kaeder C.S., Hirshman C.A.: Acute airway obstruction: A complication of aluminum tape wrapping of tracheal tubes in laser surgery. *Can. Anaesth. Soc. J.* 26:138–139, 1979.
58. Brightwell A.P.: A complication of the use of the laser in ENT surgery. *J. Laryngol. Otol.* 97:1139–1144, 1983.
59. Fried M.P.: Complications of CO_2 laser surgery of the larynx. *Laryngoscope* 93:275–278, 1983.
60. LeJune F.E. Jr., Guici C., LeTard F., et al.: Heat sink protection against lasering endotracheal cuffs. *Ann. Otol. Rhinol. Laryngol.* 91:606–607, 1982.
61. Strong M.S., Vaughan C.W., Mahler D.L., et al.: Cardiac complications of microsurgery of the larynx: Etiology, incidence and prevention. *Laryngoscope* 84:908–920, 1974.
62. Andrews A.H. Jr., Polanyi T.G., Grybauskas V.T.: General techniques and clinical considerations in laryngologic laser surgery. *Otolaryngol. Clin. North Am.* 16:793–800, 1983.
63. Alberti P.S.: The complications of CO_2 laser surgery of otolaryngology. *Acta Otolaryngol.* 91:375–381, 1981.
64. Carruth J.A.S., McKenzie A.L., Wainwright A.L.: The carbon dioxide laser: Safety aspects. *J. Laryngol. Otol.* 94:411–417, 1980.

6 Complications of CO_2 Laser Surgery of the Oral Cavity and Nasal Cavity

Robert H. Ossoff, D.M.D., M.D.

The CO_2 laser offers new and exciting possibilities for improving conventional techniques and expanding the scope of the specialty of otolaryngology–head and neck surgery. Widespread use of the CO_2 laser for treating lesions of the oral cavity, pharynx, larynx, and tracheobronchial tree has been facilitated by previous experience with the techniques of endolaryngeal microsurgery.

In the oral cavity, benign tumors can be excised or vaporized with the laser. A one-stage tongue release can be effectively performed; this procedure is helpful when rehabilitating patients following composite resection with tongue flap reconstruction.[1] Here, speech and sometimes deglutition can be improved in selected cases. Multiple areas of leukoplakia can be precisely excised or vaporized; in most instances, a graft will not be necessary to resurface the operative wound.[2] Selected superficial carcinomas can be excised with the use of the laser[3] and large recurrent or inoperable tumors can be debulked for palliation.[2] At this time, the CO_2 laser is our instrument of choice for those far-advanced cases requiring palliation.

Within the nasal cavities and paranasal sinuses, the CO_2 laser is used to treat choanal atresia,[4] hypertrophic inferior turbinates,[5] squamous papilloma, nasal polyposis, synechiae, and hereditary hemorrhagic telangiectasia.[6] For this latter condition, we believe the argon laser to be a more efficacious instrument.

ADVANTAGES OF LASER SURGERY

The greatest advantage of the CO_2 laser is precision, which allows the surgeon to make very accurate lesions. When the CO_2 laser is coupled to the operating microscope with a micromanipulator, it becomes possible to achieve surgical accuracy within 0.1 mm. The smallest spot sizes range from 0.45 mm (200-mm objective) to 0.8 mm (400-mm objective) with current technology. Most surgical procedures in the oral cavity and nasal cavity are performed using a 300-mm objective, which yields a 0.6-mm spot size. The control provided by the micromanipulator attached to the operating microscope is significantly more than is available when the laser is hand held without the advantage of magnification. The second major benefit of the CO_2 laser is hemostasis and decreased blood loss. The third major advantage of the CO_2 laser is decreased postoperative edema. A fourth advantage is decreased postoperative pain, which has been reported to be reduced or absent after using the CO_2 laser. This apparently results from the thermal sealing of nerve endings in the operative wound. Other advantages that have been attributed to the CO_2 laser include decreased postoperative scarring, uncomplicated wound healing, shorter hospitalization, simplification of many surgical techniques, and capability to use this instrument in the presence of selected coagulopathies or blood dyscrasias.

PRECAUTIONS FOR ORAL AND NASAL LASER SURGERY

Protection of the endotracheal tube from either direct or reflected laser beam irradiation is of primary importance. Should the laser beam strike an unprotected endotracheal tube carrying oxygen, ignition of the tube could result in a catastrophic, intraluminal, blowtorch-type airway fire.[7] Red rubber tubes wrapped circumferentially with reflective tape reduce the risk of intraluminal fire. For most oral cavity procedures performed under general anesthesia, nasotracheal intubation with an unwrapped red rubber endotracheal tube is used. Here, placing a saline-saturated pharyngeal pack in the oropharynx to protect the endotracheal tube from possible laser beam irradiation guards against the risk of tube fire. This pharyngeal pack will need to be moistened frequently during the procedure.

Additional precautions must be taken to provide for adequate smoke evacuation from the oral cavity and nasal cavity to allow for visualization of the operative field.

In treating lesions of the oral and nasal cavities, the laser should be attached to the operating microscope whenever possible; this allows the beam to be precisely controlled with the micromanipulator. The hand-held attachment may be an advantage when larger lesions are to be treated. The light of the newer halogen microscopes provides adequate illumination; for those microscopes with tungsten lamps, fiberoptic light bundles brought in from the side of the operative field will serve to supplement the lighting needs. The magnification provided by the operating microscope affords the surgeon the opportunity to perform close inspection of the lesion and delicate dissection of the surrounding tissue planes.

When an oral cavity lesion is found to be suitable for excision, the laser is used in the pulsed mode to outline the area of excision; this is carried through the mucous membrane. Next, traction sutures are placed; these facilitate better cutting and coagulation by the laser. Bleeding from vessels greater than 1 mm will usually need to be clamped and ligated or electrocoagulated. Frozen-section control of all margins when treating patients with a malignant neoplasm is of paramount importance. Here, the specimen should be sent to the pathologist on a specimen mount, labeled, and oriented. We have found a greater tendency for postoperative edema to occur when performing a cancer excision or tongue release in the anterior floor-of-the-mouth. In these cases, we utilize intraoperative corticosteroids (dexamethasone, 0.2 mg/kg). Most wounds in the oral cavity are left open to granulate and heal by secondary intention. Postoperative oral hygiene includes the use of one-half strength hydrogen peroxide or saline mouth washes four to six times a day until wound healing has taken place (usually 14 to 21 days).

When working in the nasal cavity, it is extremely helpful to vasoconstrict the mucous membranes with phenylephrine hydrochloride (0.25%) or vasoconstrict and topically anesthetize the mucous membranes with cocaine hydrochloride (4%) prior to beginning the procedure. A saline-saturated pharyngeal pack should be placed in the nasopharynx to protect the tissues in that area from injury. This pack also serves as a marker to aid in determining the depth of excision when working on a patient with a complete nasal obstruction such as atresia. Otologic specula are best suited to both expose the nasal cavity and protect the alar rim from accidental injury. Smoke evacuation is provided by a Rosen suction tip and additional illumination by a fiberoptic light bundle from a laryngoscope. In those cases where a lumen has been created (choanal atresia), it will be necessary to place a stent of Silastic® to maintain the lumen. In other cases where the septum and lateral wall have been denuded of mucosa, a Silastic® sheet should be placed and sutured to the septum to prevent the formation of a synechiae. These are usually left in place from ten days to two weeks. Antibiotics should be prescribed in these patients to reduce the formation of granulation tissue.

COMPLICATIONS

When the safety precautions mentioned previously have been observed, complications associated with the transoral and transoral resection of lesions using the CO_2 laser are few. Failure to provide protection to the surrounding tissues or endotracheal tube could result in accidental burns to the skin, lips, alar rim, teeth, or surrounding mucous membranes, or in a catastrophic intraluminal endotracheal tube fire (Plate 1). Postoperative edema should be minimal if proper traction has been applied during the case. Postoperative hemorrhage should not be of concern if difficult vessels were ligated or electrocoagulated as they were encountered.

Strong et al.[8] reviewed 57 cases of oral cancer managed by transoral excision with the laser; in this group of patients, there were no incidents of either postoperative bleeding or airway obstruction. In 1982, Carruth[9] reported that 25 patients had resection of tongue lesions using the CO_2 laser. Significant bleeding occurred in only one patient. Our experience with 47 patients undergoing laser surgery of the oral cavity was associated with four complications, two burns (lip and tooth) and two incidences of postoperative airway obstruction in patients who had undergone tongue release.[10] Following the successful performance of a tongue release, it is necessary to send the patient to the recovery room in the lateral decubitus position to avoid prolapse of the newly released tongue into the oropharynx causing airway obstruction. Additionally, it is advisable to extubate the patient after he or she is fully awake.

Excessive application of laser energy to a thick plate of bone in a patient with choanal atresia will produce a recurrent stenosis secondary to the necrosis of surrounding bone associated with the excessive heat absorption. Denuded mucosal surfaces on the septum and lateral nasal wall predispose the patient to the formation of a web or synechiae. This hazard should be anticipated when raw opposing surfaces are observed; here, judicious use of splints or stents will help to prevent this complication. Turbinate surgery with the CO_2 laser can produce undesirable results similar to those obtained with cryosurgery. Here, removal of only the inferior aspect of the turbinate will help to prevent such untoward results as excessive crust formation, offensive odor, mucosal drying, and recurrent epistaxis.

CONCLUSION

Although originally designed for endolaryngeal surgery, the CO_2 laser has found a unique application in disorders of the oral cavity and nasal passages. Diminished swelling, bleeding, and, especially, pain, offer advantages not found in other methods of treatment. Complications can most often be avoided by protection of the patient and the anesthetic devices.

REFERENCES

1. Liston S.L., Giordano A.: Tongue release using the CO_2 laser. *Laryngoscope* 91:1010–1011, 1981.
2. Ossoff R.H., Larlan M.S.: Laser surgery in otolaryngology, in Ballenger J.J. (ed.): *Diseases of the Nose, Throat, and Ear,* ed 13. Philadelphia, Lea & Febiger Co. In press.
3. Strong M.S., Vaughan C.W., Jako G.J., et al.: Transoral resection of cancer of the oral cavity: The role of the CO_2 laser. *Otolaryngol. Clin. North Am.* 12:207–218, 1979.
4. Healy G.B., McGill T., Jako G.J., et al.: Management of choanal atresia with the carbon dioxide laser. *Ann. Otol. Rhinol. Laryngol.* 87:658–662, 1978.
5. Mittelman H.: CO_2 laser turbinectomies for chronic, obstructive rhinitis. *Lasers Surg. Med.* 2:29–35, 1982.
6. Simpson G.T., Shapshay S.M., Vaughan C.W., et al.: Rhinologic surgery with carbon dioxide laser. *Laryngoscope* 92:412–415, 1982.
7. Ossoff R.H., Pongracic J.: The endotracheal tube problem in CO_2 laser surgery of the upper aerodigestive tract. *Symp. Proc. Laser Instit. Am.* 32:60–71, 1982.
8. Strong M.S., Vaughan C.W., Healy G.B., et al.: Transoral management of localized carcinoma of the oral cavity using the CO_2 laser. *Laryngoscope* 89:897–905, 1979.
9. Carruth J.A.S.: Resection of the tongue with the carbon dioxide laser. *J. Laryngol. Otol.* 96:529–543, 1982.
10. Ossoff R.H., Hotaling A.J., Karlan M.S., et al.: CO_2 laser in otolaryngology–head and neck surgery: A retrospective analysis of complications. *Laryngoscope* 93:1287–1289, 1983.

7 Otologic Complications of Laser Surgery

David M. Vernick, M.D.

The use of lasers in otologic surgery is still in its infancy. Almost every procedure done by conventional techniques is being tried with at least one type of laser. The advantages and disadvantages, benefits, and risks of conventional vs. laser methods are presently being reviewed to determine what, if any use lasers will play in the future of otologic surgery.

For otologic work, the laser must have many attributes (Table 7–1). The laser needs to have a beam that is small, preferably of the order of 0.1 mm. The beam should be easily and accurately focused. The beam should be able to vaporize all types of tissue, bone, tendon, and soft tissue. The beam should not affect tissue surrounding the area of work. The beam should be transportable in a fiberoptic system so that it can be used to work around corners. The laser should present no safety hazards to those using the system nor to support personnel in the immediate vicinity. The beam should be variable in power and size so that it can work on small delicate areas as well as large bone or tumor masses. It should not scatter viable cells such as squamous epithelium or tumor cells. It should not cause mutagenic or carcinogenic changes in surrounding tissues.

Unfortunately, the perfect laser system has yet to be developed for otologic surgery. It is doubtful that any single type of laser will be versatile enough to fulfill all the surgical needs mentioned above. To accomplish this, integration of several types of lasers into one microscopic delivery system will probably be necessary.

TYPES OF LASERS

The major types of medical lasers in use today (argon, CO_2, and Nd:YAG) have been discussed already in this book. Of these, only the CO_2 and argon lasers have found use in otologic surgery.[1,2] The Nd:YAG laser seems to penetrate too deeply to be of use in the ear.[2,3]

TABLE 7–1.—Desirable Features for Otologic Laser

Variable beam size down to 0.1 mm
Variable power output
Easy and accurate focus of beam
Works well on all tissues
No scatter or deep penetration
Carried via fiberoptic system
No safety hazards associated with use of laser
No mutagenic or carcinogenic properties
Does not scatter viable cells
Inexpensive, economical system

A newly developed laser using ultraviolet (UV) light may find use in otologic surgery.[4] It vaporizes tendon and bone without heating the surrounding area. Further experimental work needs to be performed prior to its use in humans. Ultraviolet light has marked mutagenic properties. Whether the UV laser will be carcinogenic in humans remains to be seen.

The argon laser system offers several distinct advantages over the present CO_2 lasers.[1] First, the wavelength of light produced is shorter. This allows for a smaller spot size and a higher power density in the beam, thus giving improved accuracy in use and a sharper "knife" to cut with. Secondly, the argon laser is visible. This visibility eliminates the uncertainty of aiming the laser beam that is present with a CO_2 laser. Thirdly, the argon laser can travel in a fiberoptic cable, whereas a CO_2 laser travels in air reflected by mirrors. This increased flexibility has yet to be exploited in otologic surgery.

The CO_2 laser may offer some advantages when dealing with large soft-tissue tumors.[1] It can vaporize large masses of tissue more quickly than the argon laser. Its benefits with acoustic tumor removal have been claimed by at least two separate groups.[5, 6] The argon laser can be used, but it does not have enough power to vaporize medium- and large-sized acoustic tumors at an acceptable pace.[7] The CO_2 laser has also been shown to perform an adequate myringotomy,[8] tympanic neurectomy, and tympanic membrane débridement.[9] For the majority of otologic surgery, however, the argon laser seems to be the better choice. For the rest of this chapter when discussing lasers, unless otherwise stated, the term will refer to the argon laser.

USES OF LASERS IN EAR SURGERY

Almost all otologic surgery done today can be and is being done without the use of lasers (Table 7–2). Therefore, the use of the laser in any proce-

TABLE 7–2.—USES OF LASERS IN EAR SURGERY

EXTERNAL CANAL AND TYMPANIC MEMBRANE	MIDDLE EAR	INNER EAR, SKULL BASE, POSTERIOR FOSSA
Current Uses		
Hemostasis	Stapedectomy	Glomus tumor removal
Granulation tissue removal	Granulation tissue & fibrous scar removal	Acoustic tumor removal
Myringotomy	Cholesteatoma removal	
Stabilization of tympanoplasty grafts	Perforating a mobile footplate	
	Sculpturing of prostheses	
Theoretical Use		
Removal of exostosis	Eustachian tube surgery	Treatment of Meniere's disease
	Obliterative otosclerosis surgery	Resections of carcinoma of temporal bone
	Congenital atresia repair	Selective vestibular ablation
	Release of malleus fixation	

dure must offer an advantage over conventional surgical techniques. These advantages might include improvement of results, reduction of operative time, reduction of postoperative recovery time, simplification of surgery, improvement of visibility, or reduction in trauma to surrounding structures. The cost of the laser system cannot be justified in our present day budgetary problems unless it can be proven to be cost effective.

Middle Ear—Myringotomy

Starting with the simplest of procedures, myringotomy, the argon laser can create a bloodless hole in the tympanic membrane.[10] Since bleeding is rarely a problem, either intraoperatively or postoperatively in blocking up the tube, this indication is borderline at best. Contrary to earlier thoughts, although the perforations look much nicer, they do not stay open any longer than perforations made with a cold knife.

Tympanoplasty

Since the laser can coagulate tissue, it can be used to stabilize tympanic membrane grafts and to weld them in place.[11] This will prevent slippage of the graft that occasionally occurs. Use of the laser can also eliminate the need for middle ear packing. This might theoretically lead to fewer middle ear adhesions. Whether or not this proves to be superior to present day packing techniques remains to be studied. The future availability of fibrin glue may prove to be superior to either method if a way to produce it without using pooled blood is developed.

Stapedotomy

In patients with otosclerosis the laser has been shown to be effective in performing stapedotomies.[12–14] The laser can perform three tasks. The first step, that of cutting the stapedius tendon, can be performed just as easily using the Belluci scissors. The second step of vaporizing the posterior crus of the stapes arch is easier and less traumatic with a laser than with crural scissors. This step weakens the superstructure and allows a better chance of fracturing the superstructure without mobilizing or dislocating the footplate. The anterior crus cannot be lasered in most ears, as the position of the stapes prevents a direct line visual access. The third step is fenestrating the footplate. Multiple laser bursts on the footplate can create a nearly circular perforation of just the correct dimensions needed prior to insertion of the piston. The procedure is atraumatic and avoids the possible suction-type injury that can occur on total footplate removal. The procedure lessens the chance of pieces of footplate falling into the vestibule. It avoids removal of too much footplate. It also lessens the chances of postoperative vertigo secondary to a perilymph fistula because the prosthesis fills the fenestra completely.

Of course if the oval window is obliterated by bone, the utility of the laser is lessened. The fenestration can be accomplished with a diamond drill as was done previously or the bone can be thinned with a drill and perforated with the laser. Lasering the entire thickness of the bone is a long and tedious task that can lead to excessive heat buildup. If the round window is obliterated with bone as well, nothing can be done even with the laser.

Revision Stapedectomy

In revision stapes surgery the argon laser has an even greater utility.[15] Middle ear adhesions can be atraumatically lysed. The old stapes prosthesis can be freed from fibrous tissue around the oval window. If the surgeon used a Gelfoam wire or fat wire, the wire can very often be removed while preserving the seal in the oval window. Removal of this seal can cause inner ear trauma if adhesions have formed between the fat or Gelfoam and the saccule or utricle. Although it is too early to tell, it is hoped that the success of revision stapes surgery can be improved from its present level to a more acceptable level (near that of primary stapedectomy) and the risks of revision surgery lessened.

Chronic Ear Surgery

In chronic ear surgery, the laser can do several things that routine techniques do with difficulty.[12] First, granulation tissue and fibrous tissue can be removed atraumatically and with minimal bleeding. Second, cholesteatoma around the ossicles can be removed from small crevices. Third, a floating footplate can be easily perforated to allow for secure ossicular reconstruction, either with a total ossicular replacement prosthesis or with a malleus-oval window wire. A prosthesis can easily be anchored to a small lasered pit in a floating footplate without risking the trauma of drilling on or near the footplate. Alternatively, a small fenestra can be lasered in the footplate to allow for passage of a piston.

Since the argon laser is precise and atraumatic it was hoped that use of the laser would allow successful reconstruction of some of the severely adhesed or tympanosclerotic middle ears. Although the ear may look good at the end of a laser operation to remove adhesions, much of the scarring reforms postoperatively. The long-term gains from such cases, therefore have been minimal. Newer techniques need to be developed to improve these results.

Eustachian Tube

Work on the eustachian tube has not been advanced with the laser. Access is only available to the two ends of the tube with our present system. Perhaps a flexible fiberoptic system could be functional in the tube to remove adhesions if an effective support could be found to allow for healing.

Acoustic Neuromas

In acoustic tumor surgery, except in small-sized tumors, the argon laser is not sufficiently powerful to be of great use. The CO_2 laser, however, offers a significant advantage in debulking of tumors, especially when the tumor is fibrous.[5] The laser eliminates much of the tugging and pulling necessary with conventional techniques. While the surgery may not be any faster, it is less traumatic. Postoperative complications should decrease as skill is developed in this surgical area.

Glomus Tumors

The argon laser has a definite role in glomus tumor surgery. Since it acts preferentially on red pigmented tissues, it can be very useful in excising the tumor. Embolization of the tumor may be necessary prior to surgery though, as the laser does not work well in the face of rapid bleeding.

Congenital Atresia

The argon laser has not found a niche as yet in surgery on congenital atresias. As in the case of a patient with an obliterated footplate from otosclerosis, the argon laser will not readily cut through thick bone without building up excessive heat and taking excessive time. Use of a drill is still the best treatment for these patients. Perhaps the UV laser will be of value in such cases if it can be proven to be safe.

Cancer of the Temporal Bone

The argon laser has not had much use in cancers of the temporal bone. Some work with preferential uptake of dyes in tumors is presently underway. Use of the laser set to a wavelength of a dye preferentially absorbed by tumor cells may make selective tumor ablation possible. Tumor might be able to be tracked as it spreads through the temporal bone and skull base.

Inner Ear

The laser has not found any utility in surgery of the inner ear. Labyrinthectomies and creation of permanent inner ear fistulas may be possible procedures under laser control. Difficulty in access to the inner ear, focusing of the laser in an underwater environment, and the manufacture of a smaller fiberoptic delivery cable are problems that await solutions. Small fiberoptic systems will need to be coupled to the microscope to permit exploration of this area.

DANGERS AND COMPLICATIONS

The argon laser is not the ultimate solution to otologic surgical problems. Its interaction with soft tissue can lead to edema for several days.[6] Its absorption by red pigment has great utility, but its use with tissues such as bone and tendon that have little or no pigment is lessened since they absorb the beam poorly. This leads to problems with cutting or vaporizing such tissues. A char may develop on bone. This slows down surgery because either the char has to be cleaned frequently or excessive heating will occur. It may be possible to apply the use of dyes or shine a ruby laser on the area of surgery to color the tissues that the laser is to vaporize. This would improve the laser selectivity and effectiveness. These alternatives have yet to be thoroughly explored.

The argon laser has to have a direct access to the tissues it is working on. At present the beam can only be directed from the microscope in a straight line. Mirrors can sometimes be used to reflect the beam inside the ear, but their accuracy is questionable and at best, variable.

Fluid or blood on tissues that are to be cut or vaporized can make the laser useless. The fluid will absorb the energy of the laser and boil away leaving the area of concern hot and uncut.

Heat can build up if long laser exposure time is used.[17] Inner ear fluids have actually boiled when exposure times have been too long. Short duration (0.1 to 0.2 second) impulses as well as careful avoidance of direct lasering into the perilymph can eliminate most of these problems.

The laser beam must be focused on the area of concern. The intensity drops markedly away from the point of focus.[18] This can be viewed as a double-edged sword. It can slow down surgery if a beam is used over larger areas. Should an impulse go off the mark, though, it can prevent serious injury to tissues not in the plane of the target.

The argon laser when used in laser stapedotomy has been shown to cause depression of the cochlear microphonic,[19,20] the compound action potential,[20,21] and the extracochlear dc potential.[22] These responses are thought to be secondary to the heat produced in fenestrating the footplate. The actual consequences of these findings seem to be limited, however. The cochlear microphonic potential recovers rapidly, leaving no long-lasting nor irreversible effects. The compound action potential takes a few seconds longer, but it as well returns back to normal. An extracochlear dc potential is produced by the impact of the laser beam on the stapes footplate. It is also probably secondary to heating of the stapes footplate. It heralds no known harmful side effects. Careful use of the laser with short exposure times of 0.1 second and resting time between each exposure will minimize, if not eliminate any consequences of heat buildup in the inner ear.

Damage to the inner ear structures has been shown to occur in animals secondary to argon, CO_2, and ruby laser irradiation.[23–26] This damage can occur with little to no damage to the overlying bone. Attempts to utilize this property to cause selective vestibular and cochlear ablation in pigeons and monkeys has been less than successful.[23,24] Scar tissue does form in the semicircular canals along with atrophy of the sensory epithelium, but the response is not predictable. Further experiments with the length and intensity of irradiation must be performed to improve these results. A middle ear procedure that would ablate vestibular function without loss of cochlear function would be a welcome advance.

Perforation of the saccule during laser stapedotomy has been documented in three of eight cat ears.[27] Since the animals were sacrificed in the immediate postoperative period, it is not known whether these cats would have been symptomatic. Certainly human patients are less vertiginous following laser stapedotomy as compared with conventional techniques. If perforations of the saccule do occur in humans, they neither produce significant postoperative vertigo, nor impair the hearing results achieved by surgery.[12]

Facial paralysis can occur if the beam is used on, or too close to, the nerve. Either direct injury or thermal injury can cause loss of facial function. Accuracy and discretion in the use of the laser can prevent this problem.

With all of the work that has been done to date, complications from the use of the laser in ear surgery are uncommon. No life-threatening side effects have been reported. No injury to the surgeon nor OR personnel have occurred when proper eye protection procedures have been followed. While occasional minor problems do occur, many of these can be eliminated by the use of good judgment by an experienced surgeon.

TIPS FOR SUCCESSFUL USE OF THE LASER IN EAR SURGERY

1. Refocus beam prior to each day's use of the laser.

2. Recalibrate beam strength daily. Small variations can and do occur from day to day. Accurate knowledge of power output means accurate estimations of cutting power.

3. Get good exposure of surgical area. You need straight line access to the target so that no reflection of the beam off of instruments occurs.

4. Work only in a dry field.

5. Suction to remove vaporized tissue. The smoke can scatter subsequent laser beams.

6. When working on bone or tendon establish a spot of char. Work outward from the area of char as the tissues will absorb the beam better.

7. Do not expect the laser to improve your speed of surgery. Especially when you start, the surgery may actually be a little longer than usual.

SET-UP FOR LASERS

Since the laser beam has to be brought into the surgical field, stationing of the laser equipment on the side of the room opposite anesthesia is preferable (Fig 7–1). Argon lasers can be transmitted along fiberoptic cables, how-

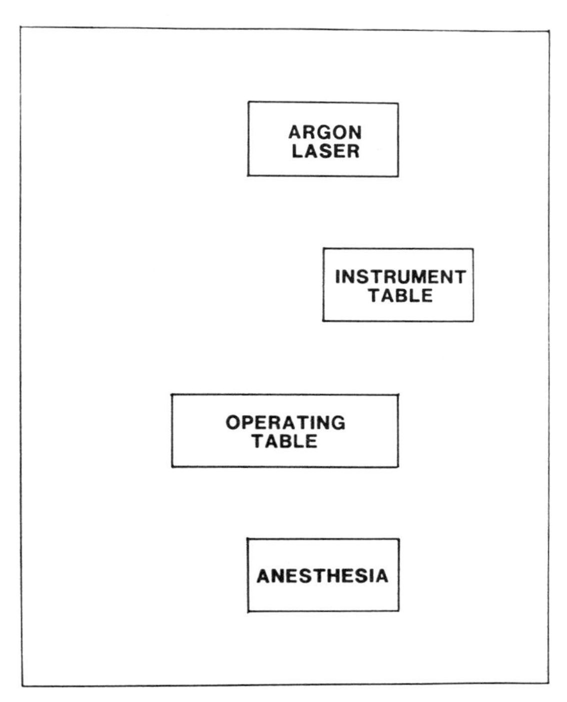

Fig 7–1. Efficient OR design for ear surgery. Instrument table can be moved depending on whether surgery is on the right or left ear.

ever, so that this requirement is flexible. One room has to be dedicated to the laser (Fig 7–2). Wherever the main instrument is set up, it must remain stable and stationary. Argon lasers break or become misaligned very easily if they are moved. They also require a water-cooling system. If possible, one microscope should also be dedicated to the laser. Since the laser can be used on almost any ear case, it should be set up and ready for every otologic procedure. Orange colored glasses for eye protection should be worn by all but the surgeon. The surgeon is protected by an orange filter that automatically flips into the microscope view when the laser is fired. Clear eye glasses that are adequate for CO_2 lasers are *not* adequate for argon laser protection.

CONCLUSIONS

Lasers are beginning to carve out a niche for themselves in otologic surgery. At present they are mainly used for middle ear procedures. Laser technol-

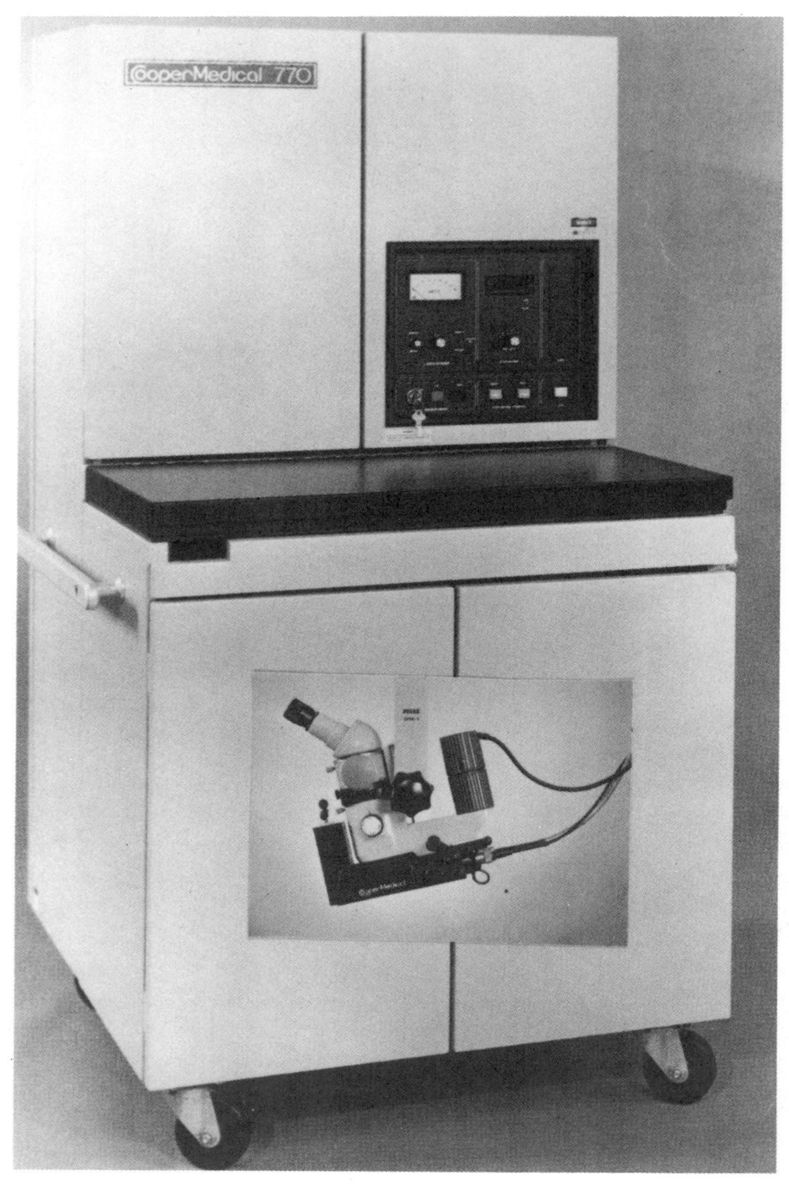

Fig 7–2. Argon laser in OR. Inset shows attachment to operating microscope.

ogy, however, is expanding very rapidly. Many of the shortcomings of present day systems should be overcome in the near future. Increased power, fiberoptic delivery, and differential tissue reaction are just a few of the advances expected. The modern otologist can expect increased advances in laser technology over the ensuing years.

REFERENCES

1. DiBartolomeo J.R.: The argon and CO_2 lasers in otolaryngology: Which one, when and why? *Laryngoscope* 26:91(pt 2), 1981.
2. Clark W., Robertson J., Gardner G.: Selective absorption and control of thermal effects: A comparison of the laser systems used in otology and neurotology. *Otolaryngol. Head Neck Surg.* 92:73–79, 1984.
3. Kelemen G., Laor Y., Klein E.: Laser induced ear damage. *Arch. Otolaryngol.* 86:21–27, 1967.
4. Present G.: Heatless laser etching. *IBM Research Highlights.* Nov 3, 1983.
5. Gardner G., Robertson J., Clark W.C.: 105 patients operated upon for cerebellopontine angle tumors: Experience using combined approach and CO_2 laser. *Laryngoscope* 93:1049–1055, 1983.
6. Glasscock M.: Personal communication.
7. Glasscock M.E. III, Jackson C., Whitaker S.: The argon laser in acoustic tumor surgery. *Laryngoscope* 91:1405–1416, 1981.
8. Lima J., Wilpizeski C.: Effectiveness of the CO_2 laser in experimental tympanic neurectomy. *Laryngoscope* 90:414–422, 1980.
9. Epley J.: Tympanic membrane debridement with the CO_2 laser. *Otolaryngol. Head Neck Surg.* 89:898–902, 1981.
10. Goode R.L.: CO_2 laser myringotomy. *Laryngoscope* 92:420–423, 1982.
11. Escudero L., Castro A., Orumond M., et al.: Argon laser in human tympanoplasty. *Arch. Otolaryngol.* 105:252–253, 1979.
12. McGee T.M.: The argon laser in surgery for chronic ear disease and otosclerosis. *Laryngoscope* 93:1177–1182, 1983.
13. Sataloff J.: Experimental use of laser in otosclerotic stapes. *Arch. Otolaryngol.* 85:58–60, 1967.
14. Perkins R.: Laser stapedotomy for otosclerosis. *Laryngoscope* 90:228–241, 1980.
15. McGee T.M.: Personal communication.
16. Gillis T., Strong S., Shapshay S., et al.: Argon laser soft tissue interaction. *Otolaryngol. Head Neck Surg.* 92:7–12, 1984.
17. Vollrath M., Schreiner C.: The effects of the argon laser on temperature within the cochlea. *Acta Otolaryngol.* 93:341–348, 1982.
18. DiBartolomeo J.R., Ellis M.: The argon laser in otology. *Laryngoscope* 90:1786–1796, 1980.
19. Vollrath M., Schreiner C.: Influence of argon laser stapedotomy on cochlear potentials: I. Alteration of cochlear microphonics (CM). *Acta Otolaryngol.* 385, 1982.

20. Vollrath M., Schreiner C.: Influence of argon laser stapedotomy on inner ear function and temperature. *Otolaryngol. Head Neck Surg.* 91:516–521, 1983.
21. Schreiner C., Vollrath M.: Effect of argon laser stapedotomy on cochlear potentials: II. Alteration of the compound action potential (CAP). *Acta Otolaryngol.* 95:47–53, 1983.
22. Vollrath M., Schreiner C.: Influence of argon laser stapedotomy on cochlear potential: III. Extracochlear recorded DC potential. *Acta Otolaryngol.* 96:49–55, 1983.
23. Stahle J., Hogberg L.: Laser and labyrinth. *Acta Otolaryngol.* 60:367–373, 1966.
24. Stahle J., Hogberg L., Engstrom B.: The laser as a tool in inner-ear surgery. *Acta Otolaryngol.* 73:27–37, 1972.
25. Wilpizeski C., Sataloff J., Doyle C., et al.: Selective vestibular ablation in monkeys by laser irradiation. *Laryngoscope* 82:1045–1058, 1972.
26. Wilpizeski C.: Experimental labyrinthotomy in monkeys by argon and carbon dioxide lasers. *Otolaryngol. Head Neck Surg.* 89:197–203, 1981.
27. Gantz B.J., Jenkins H.A., Kishimoto S., et al.: Argon laser stapedectomy. *Ann. Otol.* 91:25–26, 1982.

8 Complications of Bronchoscopic Surgery Using the Nd:YAG Laser

Stanley M. Shapshay, M.D.

The Nd:YAG laser is a relatively new medical laser that has established an important place in medical application next to the CO_2 and argon lasers. The heart of the Nd:YAG laser is a crystal composed of yttrium aluminum garnet (YAG) doped with 1% to 3% of neodymium (Nd) ions. When stimulated by a high-intensity arc lamp, this Nd:YAG crystal emits laser light with a wavelength of 1,064 nm. The Nd:YAG laser enables deeper penetration and scatter in soft tissue than either the CO_2 or argon laser. This property defines the Nd:YAG laser's primary role in medical application, which is to produce controlled coagulation of tissue. Also, its ability to achieve secure hemostasis of blood vessels up to 0.5 cm in diameter is superior to that of the other medical lasers. Unlike the CO_2 laser, the Nd:YAG laser can be used efficiently through a flexible quartz fiber, which makes it a useful endoscopic tool in bronchology, gastroenterology, and urology.

A great deal of experience with the Nd:YAG laser in bronchology has been obtained over the past years in both Europe[1,2] and the United States.[3,4] Most applications have been for palliation of obstructive tracheobronchial malignancy and for treatment of tracheal stenosis because secure hemostasis is a particularly important consideration in endoscopic therapy (Table 8–1). Unfortunately, a major difficulty in application of the Nd:YAG laser is imprecise interaction of laser and soft tissue, which makes it difficult for the endoscopist to predict depth of laser penetration. Because of dangers and complications associated with use of the Nd:YAG laser, principles for safe application and appropriate treatment of complications should be followed carefully.

TABLE 8–1.—BRONCHOSCOPIC APPLICATIONS OF THE ND:YAG LASER

Palliation of tracheobronchial malignancy
Dyspnea
Hemoptysis
Obstructive pneumonia
Secure airway before radiotherapy
Treatment of selected benign tumors and lesions
Treatment of tracheal stenosis
(in selected patients with short segments of concentric stenosis without malacia of cartilage)
Miscellaneous
Disimpaction of foreign body
Angiodysplasia
Suture granulomas
Control of bleeding after biopsy

PATIENT SELECTION

Degree of urgency of operation varies among three types of potential patients for laser surgery. Elective patients are in relatively good condition, borderline patients have major tracheobronchial obstruction but are compensating, and emergency patients have nearly total obstruction of a major airway. The first two groups should be screened carefully before laser resection. Because most patients are being treated for palliation of obstruction of an airway, hemoptysis, or obstructive pneumonia from malignancy, careful preoperative evaluation is necessary. A preoperative checklist should include review of a patient's medical history with special attention to past cardiovascular problems, drug use, and previous therapy, especially radiotherapy and surgery; blood tests, especially measurement of coagulation parameters and serum potassium levels; determination of ventilatory status by tests of blood gases, chest radiography, tomography, and computed tomography (CT) but not by bronchography, which is absolutely contraindicated because complete airway obstruction is possible; review of available biopsy specimens because such tumors as small cell carcinoma are best treated with chemotherapy and radiotherapy; and flexible bronchoscopy to determine the pathologic anatomy and presentation of the tumor. An absolute contraindication to laser bronchoscopy is extrinsic compression of an airway that is obviously beyond the scope of the laser resection.

Patients with tumor of the trachea or main stem bronchi that is observable within the airway with a visible distal lumen are the best candidates for laser resection. Patients at greater risk include those with complete bronchial obstruction or involvement of a segment longer than 4 cm; tumor of the posterior tracheal wall, which presents difficulty because of its proximity to the esophagus; and tumor of the upper lobe to which access is limited, making hemorrhage hard to control. If possible, resection of tumor obstruction before radiotherapy is preferable. After resection a patient will tolerate radiotherapy better with less risk of airway obstruction secondary to edema. Also, scarring and distortion of the airway from previous radiotherapy make laser resection more difficult. Other patients at risk are those with a vascular lesion, such as carcinoid tumor, a distal tracheal tumor with bilateral obstruction of the main bronchi, and recurrence of carinal tumor after pneumonectomy. A patient with recurrence of carinal tumor after pneumonectomy is particularly unstable under anesthesia and sensitive to hypoxemia with greater risk of cardiovascular irritability.

INSTRUMENTATION

An open rigid bronchoscope system offers maximal safety. Advantages of this system over the flexible fiberoptic bronchoscope include ventilatory control of the compromised airway; distal suction with semirigid catheters simultaneous with the laser application, which is important for hemostasis; palpation of the interface of tumor and cartilage; and rapid evacuation of fragments of tumor and debris after laser photocoagulation (Fig 8–1). The tip of the rigid bronchoscope can be used as a "cookie cutter" to separate coagulated fragments of tumor and thereby shorten the operative time for tumor resection and rapidly improve a compromised airway. The laser then can be used to vaporize the base of the tumor staying parallel to the cartilage wall.

COMPLICATIONS

Although the Nd:YAG laser has had a remarkably safe record for more than four years, it is the most powerful and perhaps the most dangerous of available medical lasers. Power output of up to 100 W can be obtained with the Nd:YAG laser at intermittent or continuous exposure. Because the power density of the Nd:YAG laser is concentrated below the surface of the tissue, as opposed to on its surface as with the CO_2 laser, an intermittent exposure setting of 1 second or less with a power setting of less than 50 W, usually 40 to 45 W, is recommended for use in bronchology.

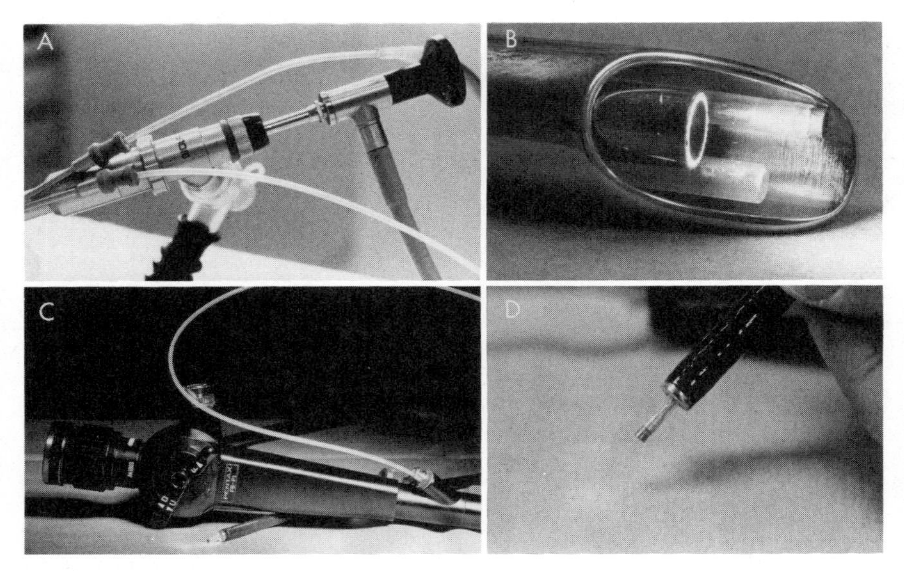

Fig 8–1. Nd:YAG fiber and semirigid suction catheter passed through rigid bronchoscope **(A and B)** and flexible fiberoptic bronchoscope **(C and D).** The suction channel is used for passage of the laser fiber. (From Beamis J.F. Jr., Shapshay S.M.: Nd-YAG laser therapy for tracheobronchial disorders. *Postgrad. Med.* 75(3):176, 1984. Used by permission.)

General hazards associated with use of the Nd:YAG laser are damage to the eye and skin of both the patient and operating room staff and ignition of surrounding combustible materials, such as surgical drapes (Fig 8–2).

Eye Safety

The eyes of the surgeon, OR personnel, and the patient should be protected carefully. Special safety goggles or glasses must be worn by all personnel in the vicinity of the Nd:YAG laser. These glasses will attenuate light specifically at 1,060 nm. Unprotected eyes may absorb the laser light primarily at the ocular fundus and cause irreparable damage. In all likelihood, eye damage will not occur if the laser is activated only when the fiber is in place inside the endoscope. The windows of the OR suite should be covered so that passersby are protected against exposure to stray laser light, although the latter is unlikely. The typical helium-neon (He-Ne) laser used as a visible red aiming light for the invisible Nd:YAG laser also can produce ocular injury, and thus the surgeon should avoid looking directly into the aiming beam. Virtually all of the He-Ne wavelength of 633 nm that strikes the eye

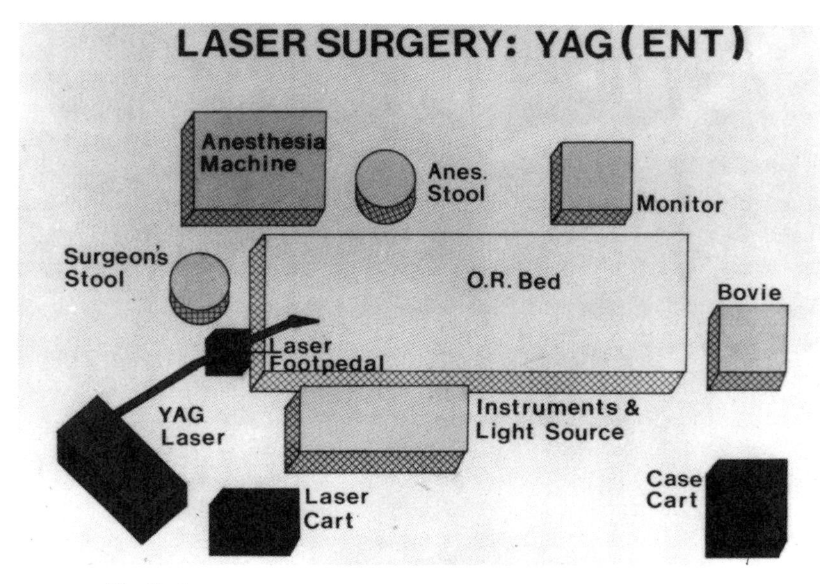

Fig 8–2. Typical OR layout for Nd:YAG otolaryngologic surgery.

is absorbed by the retina and choroid because the anterior structures are transparent. Furthermore, safety goggles do not filter out the 633-nm wavelength; if they did, the operator could not see the aiming light when it reflects from the target. Every laser sold in the United States is required by the National Center for Devices and Radiological Health of the FDA to bear a warning label with the legend, "laser aperture." No excuse exists for anyone in the laser OR to look directly into a laser aperture.

The patient's eyes are usually protected with eye goggles or by taping the eyes closed and covering them with moist cottonoids. Rumpled, heavy-gauge aluminum foil, which reflects the laser beam diffusely, affords additional protection. Moist surgical drapes are used around the operative site during external Nd:YAG laser surgery. Fortunately, superficial skin damage from the laser heals well without sequelae.

Combustion Hazards

Endotracheal Tubes.—Use of endotracheal tubes in bronchoscopic surgery is best avoided because of the risk of combustion, particularly in an oxygen-rich environment. The polyvinylchloride tube should never be used because it is rapidly punctured by a laser beam, burns readily, and produces toxic fumes and a blowtorch effect. A red rubber or silicone tube protected with self-adherent metallic reflective tape is certainly safer for the CO_2 laser but, again, is best avoided when using the Nd:YAG laser. External taping of the endotracheal tube does not protect the internal wall from combustion when using the laser inside the endotracheal tube.

Bronchoscopic Fire.—Ignition of the sheath of the flexible fiberoptic bronchoscope can cause fire.[5] This risk is increased if a high-power setting, greater than 50 W, is used in an oxygen-rich environment (greater than 50%). The sheath of the bronchoscope or the endotracheal tube is at risk, and the response to combustion should be prompt removal of flammable materials. Inspection for tracheobronchial burns and respiratory support should follow an accident, and the patient should be treated with antibiotics and steroids to diminish the inflammatory response and decrease the possibility of scarring.

Strict adherence to proper bronchoscopic technique will, of course, diminish the risk of combustion. Flammable materials within the laser bronchoscope are the laser fiber itself and plastic suction materials, so the laser fiber should be maintained free of debris at all times, and any plastic materials should be kept proximal to the fiber if possible.

Perforation of the Tracheobronchial Tree

The risk of tracheobronchial perforation with the Nd:YAG laser is certainly greater than with the CO_2 or argon laser. The depth of the Nd:YAG laser penetration and scatter is considerably greater than that of argon and CO_2 lasers and less predictable in its effect (Table 8–2). In soft tissue the Nd:YAG laser has the potential for strong, forward scattering. The point of maximum histologic power density is, therefore, not at the irradiated surface. The

TABLE 8–2.—Comparative Absorption and Scatter of Nd:YAG, CO_2, and Argon Lasers*

LASER	WAVELENGTH (μ)	ABSORPTION†	SCATTER†
Nd:YAG	1.06	77 mm^{-1}	0
CO_2	10.6	0.23 cm^{-1}	21 cm^{-1}
Argon	0.5	0.03 cm^{-1}	>3 cm^{-1}

*Reproduced from Fisher J.C.: *Some Fundamental Physical Considerations Relating to Safety and Efficacy of Surgical Lasers.* Sudbury, Mass. Cavitron Corporation, 1978, with permission.

†The coefficients of absorption and scattering are for water.

power density may be several millimeters below the surface, particularly with pale-colored tissue. Laser irradiation at continued high power, greater than 40 W, causes explosive rupture of the tissue—the so-called popcorn effect. The surgeon may see a blanching of the surface of the tissue followed by charring before explosion of the tissue takes place. Cautious intermittent Nd:YAG laser irradiation with less than 50 W of power is highly advisable during endoscopy. The Nd:YAG laser fiber should always be used parallel and never perpendicular to the tracheobronchial wall. The tip of the rigid bronchoscope is a useful palpating device to help determine the tracheal cartilage-tumor interface. This is not possible with the flexible fiberoptic bronchoscope.

Hemorrhage

Persistent uncontrolled bleeding in the tracheobronchial tree, regardless of its rate, may lead to life-threatening hypoxemia. Tracheal hemorrhage represents the most dangerous situation because the distal airway may be flooded quickly. Cessation of tumor resection and immediate hemostasis are imperative. The hemorrhage usually can be controlled by passing the ventilatory bronchoscope distally and achieving tamponade with it. Distal cleansing of the airway and ventilation are the immediate concerns followed by attention to the tumor site. Two semirigid suction catheters passed through the rigid bronchoscope are used to maintain a dry operative field while the laser is used at coagulating power of 30 to 40 W with the fiber about 2 cm away from the target tissue.[6] Coagulation should begin circumferentially around the bleeding site and move in finally to the bleeding area itself. Massive bronchial hemorrhage necessitates placement of the patient in a lateral position with the healthy lung uppermost. In this safety position the ventilatory bronchoscope is used to evacuate blood and secretions and to achieve patency.

Perforation of a major blood vessel, such as the left pulmonary artery, usually has catastrophic consequences. As most patients treated have incurable cancer, heroic measures should not be undertaken. Fortunately, this complication has been rare.[3]

Hypoxemia

The major causes of death during or after laser resection are perforation and hypoxemia. The grave danger of hemorrhage is that it results in hypoxemia, death by exsanguination being rare. Hypoxemia also can arise from a collection of secretions and debris or from anesthetically induced respiratory depression. If uncorrected, hypoxemia leads to cardiovascular complications, including, in order of increasing seriousness, arrhythmia, bradycardia, myocardial infarction, and cardiac arrest.

The anesthetic and intraoperative ventilatory technique is particularly important in prevention of hypoxemia. General anesthesia with spontaneous ventilatory technique is the preferred method for patients with obstruction of a major airway. Intravenous administration of narcotics supplemented by local, topical anesthesia is usually sufficient. On occasion, assisted ventilatory technique is necessary with the application of positive pressure through the ventilatory side arm. A Venturi technique also may be used but carries the risk of pneumothorax and blowing debris distally into the lungs. Constant monitoring of oxygen saturation by an ear oximeter and frequent monitoring of blood gases are important in high-risk patients. Adequate ventilation and frequent tracheobronchial toilet should be the endoscopist's constant preoccupations during the laser procedure. Should the oxygen saturation fall or cardiac irregularity occur, immediate attention to the distal or opposite healthy airway is mandatory.

POSTOPERATIVE COMPLICATIONS

The postoperative period is critical. In our experience,[6] most fatal complications occurred from delayed cardiovascular sequelae related to hypoxemia. Should a patient show signs of hypoxemia in the recovery room despite oxygen therapy, bronchoscopy should be performed immediately. Routine chest radiography is used to rule out collapse of the lung or pneumothorax and pulmonary edema.

The main postoperative complications are cardiovascular sequelae and hypoxemia related to retained secretions or respiratory depression induced by excessive anesthesia; secondary hemorrhage from loosened eschar or inadequate coagulation; perforation from delayed tissue necrosis resulting in fatal sequelae, such as mediastinitis or tracheobronchial fistula; and infection or pneumonia or both after atelectasis or retained secretions. The last is best avoided by a thorough laser resection and intraoperative tracheobronchial toilet. Prophylactic antibiotics are not necessary and are best avoided.

COMPLICATION RATE WITH Nd:YAG LASER BRONCHOSCOPY

Endobronchial resection with the Nd:YAG laser is a high-risk therapy to be used for high-risk patients. Because these patients are usually treated to palliate the symptoms of obstruction by a malignancy, the complication rate must be low to justify laser surgery. Complication risk has been analyzed[6] in a large combined series of patients from four medical centers in Europe and the United States in whom the same techniques of Nd:YAG laser resection were used. A total of 1,503 laser treatments was performed on 839 patients; in 1,156 patients general anesthesia with a rigid bronchoscopic technique was used (Table 8–3). All complications whether related to anesthesia or to the laser treatment were considered together because separation was impossible. Six deaths occurred in this large series, and all were related to hypoxemia, which can result from excessive anesthesia or from bleeding and retained secretions. No perforations, fires, or major arterial catastrophic hemorrhages occurred. The latter complications were avoided by preventive measures as described earlier.

TRAINING AND PREPARATION OF THE LASER ENDOSCOPIST

The laser endoscopist should be skilled in techniques of both rigid and flexible bronchoscopy and familiar with the varieties of tracheobronchial pathology and their natural history. A thorough knowledge of basic laser physics and of the interaction between laser and soft tissue is mandatory. At the Lahey Clinic Medical Center at least one certified course with hands-on experience in the laboratory is required for practice of laser endoscopy. In addition, the endoscopist should visit an established laser unit and observe

TABLE 8–3.—Immediate and Delayed Complications in 1,503 Nd:YAG Laser Bronchoscopies

Complications	No. Patients	
Immediate		
Cardiovascular		7
Severe bradycardia	3	
Cardiac arrest	2	
Circulatory collapse	2	
Hemorrhage (>200 ml)		14
Pneumothorax	3	
Delayed		
Cardiovascular		8
Anoxia	3 (2 deaths)	
Circulatory collapse	2	
Cardiac arrest	1 (1 death)	
Infarction	2 (2 deaths)	
Hemorrhage		2 (2 deaths)

clinical applications. If possible, the candidate's first four laser endoscopies are observed by a staff endoscopist with experience in the use of the laser. A clinical protocol approved by the Lahey Clinic's Institutional Review Board must be submitted before the technique may be used clinically. A laser subcommittee of the surgical administrative committee gives final accreditation and approval of the applicant's training. This subcommittee also keeps records of all laser operations performed and their results and complications. As the Nd:YAG laser has not at this time been approved by the FDA, all results must be reported also to the sponsoring laser manufacturer that holds the investigational device exemption.

CONCLUSIONS

The Nd:YAG laser has become our treatment of choice for the difficult problem of palliation of symptoms of obstructive tracheobronchial malignancy and for selected patients with tracheal stenosis and benign pathology. This laser is safe when used by an endoscopist skilled in laser technique. The importance of careful patient selection and a close working relationship with an experienced anesthesiologist cannot be overemphasized.

REFERENCES

1. Toty L., Personne C., Colchen A., et al.: Bronchoscopic management of tracheal lesions using the neodymium yttrium aluminium garnet laser. *Thorax* 36:175–178, 1981.
2. Dumon J.F., Reboud E., Garbe L., et al.: Treatment of tracheobronchial lesions by laser photoresection. *Chest* 81:278–284, 1982.
3. McDougall J.C., Cortese D.A.: Neodymium-YAG laser therapy of malignant airway obstruction: A preliminary report. *Mayo Clin. Proc.* 58:35–39, 1983.
4. Shapshay S.M., Dumon J.F., Beamis J.F. Jr.: Endoscopic treatment of tracheobronchial malignancy: Experience with Nd-YAG and CO_2 lasers in 506 operations. *Otolaryngol. Head Neck Surg.,* 93:205–210, 1985.
5. Casey K.R., Fairfax W.R., Smith S.J., et al.: Intratracheal fire ignited by the Nd-YAG laser during treatment of tracheal stenosis. *Chest* 84:295–296, 1983.
6. Dumon J.F., Shapshay S.M., Bourcereau J., et al.: Principles for safety in application of Nd-YAG laser in bronchology. *Chest,* 86:163–168, 1984.

9 Complications of Argon Laser Surgery for Skin Lesions

by Joel M. Noe, M.D.

Argon is the gas that provides the lasing media that is the basis for this type of laser. Historically, it was the argon laser that replaced the ruby laser for the treatment of vascular lesions of the skin. Although the argon laser has six different wavelengths, more than 80% of its energy output is at 488 and 514.5 mm. These wavelengths seem to have preferential absorption by hemoglobin (absorption peaks at 420, 542, and 577 mm) and relatively poor absorption in nonpigmented tissues. It is these characteristics that have been exploited in the development of lasers for the destruction of vascular and pigmented tissues.[1] Simply put, the argon laser is useful in treating superficial vascular lesions such as port wine stains (PWS), telangiectasias, and angiomas, because the blue-green light is selectively absorbed by the red-purple oxygenated hemoglobin in the superficial dermal ectatic vessels. The light energy is transformed into heat, thermal damage ensues, the vessels thrombose, and the vascular lesion lightens or disappears.[2]

In reality, however, the skin is not an ideal optical medium. Argon light is not truly monochromatic, and the interaction of this light and oxygenated hemoglobin is not fully understood. It is presumed that the direct mechanism involves the absorption of laser radiation by intravascular hemoglobin which, in turn, results in endothelial damage to the vessel wall and subsequent thrombosis. However, the heat generated also causes less specific tissue coagulation. There is nonspecific epidermal and upper dermal necrosis and subsequent fibrosis.[3] The latter may be necessary to lighten the vascular lesion and to prevent vessels from recannalizing, but also results in a nonspecific tissue coagulation and subsequent fibrosis that contributes to the complications of scarring. The relative specificity of the argon laser–hemoglobin interaction and its precise mode of inducing improvement in clinical lesions remain to be defined more clearly.

APPLICATIONS

Port wine stains represent one type of congenital malformation involving mature capillaries.[4] These "hemangioma" are members of a larger group of congenital lesions termed *nevus flammeus,* which commonly involve the forehead, face, occiput, and the nuchal regions, and are present in 75% of newborns.[5,6] At birth, they are uniformly macular, pink to red, and most disappear by the end of the first year. Port wine stains represent those nevi flammeus that persist into childhood and adult life (see Plate 2). Pathogenically, they represent an increased number of vessels in the superficial dermis, which become progressively ectatic during a person's lifetime. The color of the PWS is stable in certain patients, while in others it changes, correlating with this progressive ectasia, darkening with time from pink to red to purple. Likewise, the surface may change from smooth to irregular to the classic (cobblestone) pattern. Studies have shown an incidence of less than 1% of the population develop PWS, which may understate the true frequency for a number of reasons.[7,8] Often patients have stated that the PWS was not visible at birth. Given the relative anemic state and the erythematous condition of the skin of the neonate, one can understand how the PWS may not be appreciated at the time of birth, thus understating any statistics based on birth records or neonatal physical examination.

Telangiectasias are permanent dilatations of capillaries that are usually macular and nonpulsatile. They usually, but not always, disappear with the pressure of a glass slide. There are a number of telangiectatic lesions that commonly involve the facial skin, including rosacea, actinic ectasia, spider ectasia, telangiectatic mats, as well as a number of telangiectatic syndromes.

The postrhinoplasty "red nose" syndrome (PRRNS) refers to a complication infrequently seen after rhinoplasty[9] (see Plate 3). A "red" blush or multiple telangiectasias appear on the nasal dorsum. Usually, a large dorsal hump has been removed. Classically, the patient is a fair-skinned person who sunburns easily, tans poorly, and has had a large amount of sun exposure on the nose. The etiology is unclear, but may represent either the worsening of a preexisting condition or a secondary effect of the nasal surgery or trauma.

SURGICAL TECHNIQUES

In the first session, history, physical examination, and photographs are obtained. A test patch is used, which has the advantage of allowing the patient and family to assess the result prior to committing themselves to treating the whole lesion. The medical and nursing staff has a chance, likewise, to evaluate not only the potential result of the treatment, but also the response of the patient and family to that result prior to proceeding. A small 2-mm punch biopsy specimen of a representative section next to the test patch is obtained, the result of which is helpful when predicting the response. Essentially, the larger the vessel, the more full it is with red blood cells (RBCs), the more superficial it is, the better the response that will be noted in terms of lightening, smoothing, and flattening of the lesion. The test patch and biopsy, however, are limited to the extent that the lesion is homogenous. Noe et al. have shown that one can predict the result on the basis of the color of the lesion, the age of the patient, and the biopsy specimen.[10]

The edges of the lesion are marked by a pen to facilitate visualization by the surgeon when glasses are later applied. Noninvolved areas are also marked, as there is no need to treat these areas.

Local anesthesia is used.[11] Two percent xylocaine without epinephrine is used to maximize vessel dilatation. One should not place the needle within the lesion for fear of puncturing the vessels, releasing the needed RBCs. Therefore, the anesthetic should be applied at a distance from the lesion.

The room is closed and sealed, there should be no way for light to enter or leave the room. The door should be closed so that no one can either open it from the outside or look through it or any window. The room should be marked with suitable signs and lights on the outside of the door warning that the laser is in use. Everyone—the patient, nurses, physician and family—wears protective glasses.

The surgeon checks first the quality and contour of the light beam, making corrections where appropriate. Second, a power meter, separate from the machine, is used to verify the control module readings as the tissue levels are obviously much more important than readings obtained from within the machine.

Gilchrest et al.[12] have shown that applying ice to the skin prior to treatment may protect the overlying epidermis from injury caused by the argon laser.

The continuous mode is used. The lowest power density that will cause whitening of the tissues, and depression if the lesion is elevated, is used. The rate of movement of the light beam across the lesion is a function of the first appearance of whitening of the lesions. The edges are "feathered" to minimize depressions or furrows.

It is best to wait at least four months to evaluate the test patch, which is graded on the basis of lightening, flattening, and presence or absence of scarring (Plate 4).

Preoperative and postoperative advice is given verbally and in writing.[13] (See Boston's Beth Israel [BIH] Hospital Nurse's Sheet.) Prior to treatment, the patient is advised not to take any aspirin or aspirin-containing medications, to minimize the chance of bleeding. Likewise, the patient is advised to minimize any sun exposure as the erythematous response could absorb the laser light. Postoperatively, the patient is advised to keep his or her head elevated. Soap and water is used, and occasionally, bacitracin for the first few days. We have found no need to use any parenteral antibiotics. The dressings that are used are nonadherent and occlusive to expedite the rate of epithelialization.

COMPLICATIONS—THEIR MANAGEMENT AND AVOIDANCE

Port Wine Stains

No vessel constrictor such as epinephrine is used in an attempt to maximize the amount of vessel dilatation. Port wine stains are vascular lesions in the head and neck area. In addition, if there is an arterial-venous component, there is an additional factor that contributes to an increase in the rate of perfusion. Large areas may be treated on one procedure. All these factors increase the chance of xylocaine toxic reactions. Five to 7 mg/kg of body weight is the toxic level, and should not be exceeded given the above factors.

The local anesthetic is used for both anesthesia and for maximizing the degree of dilatation. If the needle punctures the vessels that are treated, RBCs leak out, the vessels collapse, and there is no chromophore to absorb the blue-green light of the argon laser. Hence, it is best to place the needle at a distance from the area to be treated. With smaller lesions such as telangiectasias and cherry angiomas, it may be best not to use a local anesthetic at all, for fear of damaging the vessel.

Scarring is noted in a certain segment of the population after argon laser treatment. Two types of scars are noted: a hypertrophic scar seen in the head and neck area, in particular around the lips (Plate 5), and an atrophic type of scar noted by the "cigarette-paper" quality of the skin. Dixon et al.[14] noted a 38% incidence of hypertrophic scarring when treating patients under the age of 12 years.

An increased incidence of scarring in all patients is noted when the upper lip is treated. Often there is a family history of excessive scarring. Patients with an olive complexion are noted to scar more often. I feel strongly that until our knowledge and technology have increased, we should not treat children under the age of 12 years.

The lowest amount of energy that results in lightening of the lesion should be used. The wound care should be directed to minimize any chance of infection, as this encourages scarring (Fig 9–1). Occlusive dressings maximize the rate of epithelialization. In the areas around the mouth a low energy level plus pressure and minimal motion posttreatment may all be helpful to reduce the incidence of scarring. The use of ice prior to treatment protects the epidermis and minimizes the "cigarette-paper" quality of the skin otherwise noted.[15]

No patient should be treated, nor should anyone be in the room when the laser is on, unless he or she wears protective lenses.

Simple wound care consisting of soap, water, elevation and topical antibiotics, such as bacitracin, and the fact that the majority of these PWS are treated in the head and neck area, have resulted in an incidence of infection less than 0.05%.

Occasionally, especially when smaller areas are treated, one notices a definite depression or step-off. By using a "feathering" technique, i.e., a gradual change in contour at the edges, one can minimize this problem of depression in the contour.

Patients are instructed not to ingest any aspirin or aspirin-containing compound two weeks before treatment and two weeks following treatment. The patient is instructed in the use of simple compression for five minutes by the clock should there be any bleeding in this lesion.

Telangiectasias, Cherry Angiomas

These lesions can be treated in a manner very similar to that of the PWS.[16] Essentially, the lesion is marked out prior to treatment with a skin marking pen. The "feathering" technique is used to minimize any furrows or depressions. Especially in thick sebaceous skin, such as on the tip of the nose, 1 to 2 mm of the surrounding, noninvolved area is treated as well to minimize any sharp drop-offs of treated vs. nontreated skin. Local anesthesia is not used, so that no needle can puncture the vessel. The patient is prepared by shining the laser light on the dorsum of his or her hands so that he or she can understand the type of discomfort that will be encountered on the face.

Venous Lakes—Lips

Enough power density is used to get depression and whitening. The lesion is marked out with a skin marking pen, and then local anesthesia is used. The lesion is treated much like the PWS, but often the lesion must be treated at three-week intervals to get the desired result.

Your Doctor ______________________ Your Nurse ______________________
Phone number ______________________

Beth Israel Hospital, Boston, Mass., Nursing Recommendations

Argon Laser Program

What To Expect After Laser Treatment
The following information will explain what happens after the laser has been applied to an area of your skin:
- In the first few weeks the treated skin may "weep" and then a scab may form. (Some people will heal without forming a scab.)
- After the scab falls off, the treated area may look red. This is *expected.* It *does not* mean that the treatment did not work.
- The local anesthetic, xylocaine, plus the laser treatment, may leave the treated area swollen for the next several hours or even days. If the area treated was near your eyes, your eyelids may become swollen.
- It may take from two (2) to nine (9) months for this area to lighten in color. Once this process has begun, the skin color will continue to lighten for the next year.

How To Care for Your Treated Area
In case of swelling:
- Sleep with your head elevated on several pillows to decrease facial swelling.
- Ice may decrease swelling of your eyelids if used soon after treatment and for 24 hours thereafter.
- Forced "winking" of your eyes helps decrease swelling in eyelid muscles.
- An eye patch may be worn for several days.

Skin care *until* "weeping" stops and/or a scab forms:
- Wash the area gently three (3) times a day with Dial soap and rinse well with water.
- Gently pat dry and apply a thin layer of Bacitracin ointment over the area.
- After each washing, cover the area with a clean Telfa dressing or plastic strips (such as Band-Aids).
  Note: Remove dressings carefully. Do not pull the dressing off if it is sticking to the area. Instead, soak the dressing with water until it comes off easily.

Skin care *after* "weeping" stops and/or scab forms:
- Continue to keep area clean using soap and water. Ointment and dressings are no longer necessary.
- You may apply make-up on the treated area only *after* the scab has *fallen off.* This may take two weeks, however waiting to apply make-up reduces the risk of infection.
- When the area is completely healed (which may take up to three weeks), you may resume shaving.
- You may swim in clean water. Remember to wash with soap and water after swimming.

What To Avoid Before and After Laser Treatment
Avoid direct sun exposure:
- Treated skin may be overly sensitive to the sun. The laser-treated area should not be exposed directly to the sun for ten (10) weeks after treatment. A sunscreen containing Paba is recommended.
- Avoid direct sun exposure to any area of skin that will be treated with laser for three (3) weeks prior to the treatment. Sunburn, which causes redness of the superficial skin, many absorb the laser and thereby decrease the effectiveness of the treatment.
- In order to evaluate the laser's effectiveness, your skin must not be sun burned. Avoid direct sun exposure to the treated area for three (3) weeks before an evaluation visit.

(continued)

Avoid aspirin products before treatments:

- Aspirin or aspirin-containing products (Bufferin, Anacin, Excedrin, Dristan, etc.) *must be* avoided for seven (7) days before your next treatment. Aspirin containing products can prolong bleeding.
- Tylenol can be substituted for relief of discomfort.

Please call with any questions or concerns. We look forward to assisting you.

Fig 9–1. Information sheet for patients.

Postrhinoplasty "Red Nose" Syndrome

As noted above, this is defined as a red blush or telangiectatic mass on the dorsum of the nose following nasal surgery or trauma. Sometimes the patient has some preexisting condition that is evidence of sensitivity to the sun, and often has had excessive actinic ray exposure following surgery or trauma. When these lesions are biopsied, multiple ectatic vessels in the superficial dermis are noted. Prior to nasal surgery, patients should be advised to minimize sun exposure postoperatively. The PRRNS lesion, being similar to the vascular lesions noted above (macular in nature and consisting of superficial ectatic vessels) is treated in the identical manner. Local anesthesia is used.

SUMMARY

The PWS serves as an excellent model for the interaction between the blue-green light of the argon laser and red hemoglobin molecules seen in vascular anomalies of the superficial cutaneous surface.[17] The same technique that is used to treat the PWS can be applied to treat other superficial vascular anomalies such as telangiectasias, cherry angiomas, venous lakes, and postrhinoplasty "red noses." The complications seen are slightly different: hypertrophic scars and atrophic skin are more commonly seen with PWS and depressions or furrows are more commonly seen with telangiectasias.

REFERENCES

1. Glover J.L., Bendick P.J., Link W.J.: The use of thermal knives in surgery: Electrosurgery, lasers, plasma scalpel. *Curr. Probl. Surg.* 15:1–78, 1978.
2. Arndt K.A., Noe J.M.: Lasers in dermatology. *Arch. Dermatol.* 118:293–295, 1982.
3. Finley J., Barsky S., Geer D., et al.: Healing of port wine stains after argon laser surgery. *Arch. Dermatol.* 117:486–489, 1981.
4. Barsky S., Rosen S., Geer D., et al.: The nature and evolution of port wine stains: A computer assisted study. *J. Invest. Dermatol.* 74:154–157, 1980.

5. Caro W.H.: Tumors of the skin, in Moschella, S., Pillsbury D., Hurley H. (eds.): *Dermatology*. Philadelphia, W.B. Saunders Co., 1975, pp 1323–1406.
6. Miescher G.: Uber plane Angiome (Naevi hyperaemici). *Dermatologica* 106:176–183, 1953.
7. Pratt A.G.: Birthmarks in infants. *Arch. Dermatol.* 67:302, 1953.
8. Jacobs A.H., Walton R.G.: The incidence of birthmarks in the neonate. *Pediatrics* 58:218, 1976.
9. Noe J., Arndt K.A., Finley J., et al.: The postrhinoplasty "red nose": Differential diagnosis and treatment by laser. *J. Plast. Reconstr. Surg.* 67:661–664, 1981.
10. Noe J.M.: Predictive value of age, color, and biopsy on argon laser therapy of port wine stains, in Arndt K.A., Noe J.M., Rosen S. (eds.): *Cutaneous Laser Therapy: Principles and Methods.* New York, John Wiley & Sons, 1983.
11. Arndt K.A., Burton C., Noe J.M.: Minimizing the pain of local anesthesia. *Plast. Reconstr. Surg.* 72-5:676–679, 1983.
12. Gilchrest B.A., Rosen S., Noe J.M.: Chilling port wine stains improves the response to argon laser therapy. *J. Plast. Reconstr. Surg.* 69:278–283, 1982.
13. Larrow L., Noe J.M.: Care of the patient with a port wine stain hemangioma. *Am. J. Nursing* 82-5:786–790, 1982.
14. Dixon J.A., Huether S., Rotering R.: Hypertrophic scarring in argon laser treatment of port wine stains. *Plast. Reconstr. Surg.* 73-5:770–778, 1984.
15. Gilchrest B.A., Rosen S., Noe J.M.: Chilling port wine stains improves the response to argon laser therapy. *J. Plast. Reconstr. Surg.* 69:278–283, 1982.
16. Arndt K.A.: Argon laser therapy of small cutaneous vascular lesions. *Arch. Dermatol.* 118:220–224, 1982.
17. Arndt K.A., Noe J.M., Rosen S. (eds.): *Cutaneous Laser Therapy: Principles and Methods.* New York, John Wiley & Sons, 1983.

10 Complications of CO_2 Laser Surgery in Children

Gerald B. Healy, M.D.

The use of lasers in the treatment of disorders of the head and neck began in 1971, and it soon became apparent that this would be an important therapeutic modality.[1] A few years after its introduction, reports suggested that this would become valuable as well in the treatment of disorders of the pediatric aerodigestive tract. As in all surgical techniques, however, complications may arise, especially if appropriate precautions are not taken. Several reports of complications unique to the use of the CO_2 laser have appeared in the literature.[2–4] Pediatric patients may well be at the highest risk for complications due to the smallness of the structures being treated. Therefore, it is imperative that all appropriate precautions be taken to ensure as low a complication rate as possible.

At this time the primary laser instrument used in pediatrics is the CO_2 laser. Ion lasers and solid state lasers have not demonstrated a significant use in the pediatric upper airway.

Major complications may involve either the patient or OR personnel and may be related to either anesthesia or the instrument employed in the procedure.

PEDIATRIC ANESTHESIA COMPLICATIONS

All nonmetallic materials, even though they do not contain water, will absorb CO_2 laser energy to a varying degree. The rapid conversion of this energy to heat induces melting or even ignition. Metallic surfaces reflect CO_2 laser energy, and therefore, precautions must be taken to prevent reflection of radiation onto any structures that may surround the metallic surface.

It is apparent that anesthesia delivery systems present the single greatest hazard in CO_2 laser surgery in pediatrics. The use of an unprotected plastic or polyvinylchloride endotracheal tube presents the most hazardous of delivery systems (Fig 10–1). If this type of tube is accidentally struck by the laser beam, penetration and ignition are almost instantaneous. Inasmuch as an oxygen-enriched atmosphere is already present in general anesthesia, a major fire is almost a certainty. The fire may be due either to direct impact of the laser on the tube or even to the inhalation of flaming tissue into the tip of the endotracheal tube (Fig 10–2). Fires involving an inflated cuff are usually not a problem in pediatrics inasmuch as cuffed tubes are not frequently employed.

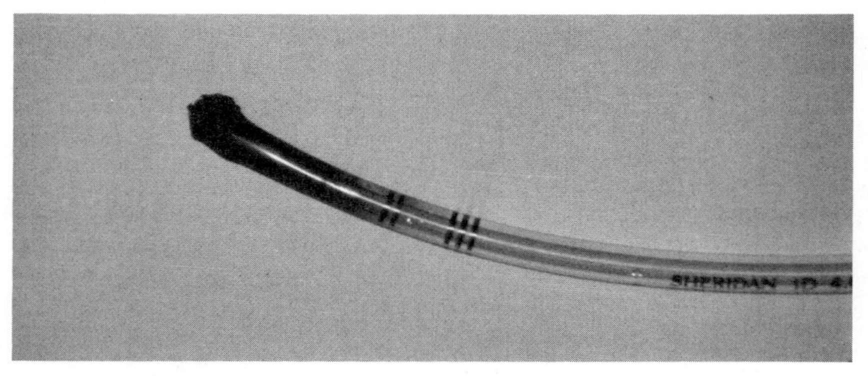

Fig 10–1. Unprotected polyvinylchloride tube. This type tube should never be used for laser surgery of the airway.

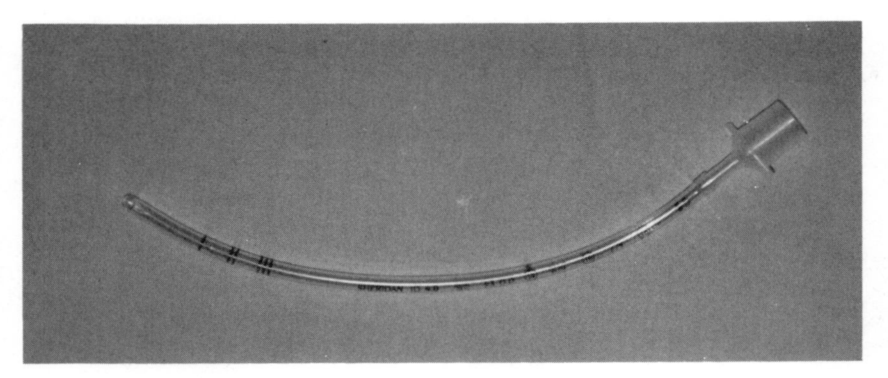

Fig 10–2. Burned polyvinyl tube secondary to aspiration of burning tissue at distal end.

It has been our experience that if one wishes to employ an endotracheal tube during laser surgery, then the use of a red rubber tube wrapped with a metallic tape seems to provide the most desirable delivery system. The tube must be carefully wrapped so that the metallic tape is tightly adherent and correctly overlapped. Before wrapping, the tube should be cleaned with acetone and coated with benzoin to provide a satisfactory adhesive surface for the tape. A sharp bevel is cut at the beginning of the tape to eliminate any free edge that could cause the tape to unravel from the tube. Wrapping is continued so that at least 6 to 10 cm of the most distal portion of the tube is covered. The tape should be overlapped at least one third to one half of its width at each consecutive turn and enough tension should be applied so that the tape does not buckle or wrinkle as it is wound (Fig 10–3). Such tubes may be sterilized with ethylene oxide and thus the tube may be prewrapped, sterilized, and stored. All tubes should be inspected before and after their use for possible damage or gaps in the reflective surface.

Reflective tapes are available that are nonmetallic and these tapes usually are of mylar film that has been impregnated with aluminum. They will not reflect CO_2 laser energy and thus should never be used for wrapping tubes, as they present an enormous fire hazard. If the surgeon is uncertain, he or she must test the tape to be used before wrapping the endotracheal tube.[4]

In most pediatric patients with laryngeal abnormalities, an indwelling

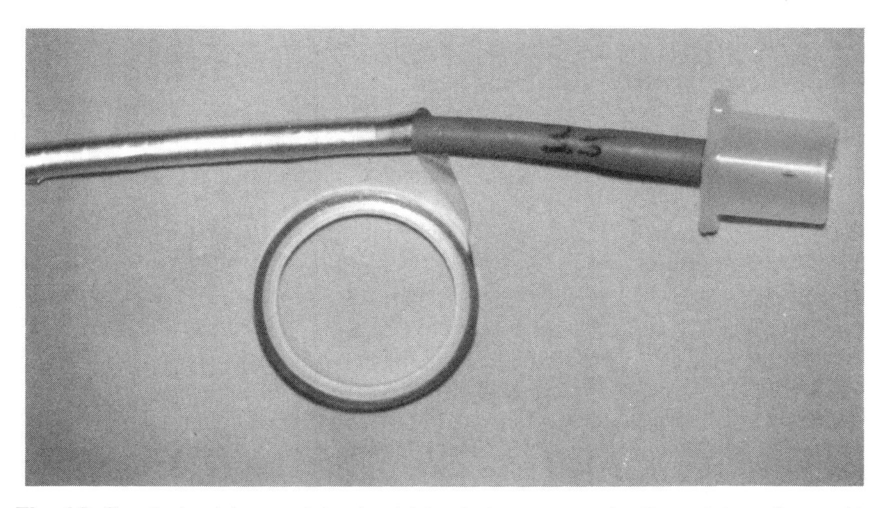

Fig 10–3. Red rubber endotracheal tube being wrapped with metal nonflammable tape.

endotracheal tube severely impairs the surgeon's ability to visualize and treat the lesion with the CO_2 laser. Therefore, it is more desirable to remove the tube and ventilate the patient by an alternative means until surgery is completed. This also significantly reduces fire hazard as combustible material is removed from the airway as well.

Venturi ventilation, jet injection techniques, and insufflation provide such an alternative. All of these modalities have potential complications associated with them and therefore should not be used without proper training and precaution.

Venturi ventilation is an extremely satisfactory alternative to intubation if carefully utilized. Proper selection and placement of the Venturi needle determine the effectiveness of the system.[5] In these cases the patient is initially intubated and positioned. After CO_2 laser apparatus has been brought into place, the patient is given an IV paralytic agent to prevent motion of the vocal cords and the endotracheal tube is removed. The Venturi apparatus, which has been previously placed on the laryngoscope, is then utilized for ventilation. One must be extremely careful, however, that the pressure settings are appropriate according to the size and weight of the patient. Only enough pressure should be used to produce slight visible chest motion and adequate bilateral breath sounds. This may vary according to the size and age of the child.

Pneumomediastinum and pneumothorax can occur if this system is not properly applied. (Fig 10–4). Gastric distention and regurgitation, as well as hypercarbia, may also be induced if care is not taken. A nasogastric tube may be passed at the start of the procedure to minimize gastric distention. Hypercarbia should not be a problem if adequate ventilation is undertaken.

Jet injection techniques, where catheters are placed below the level of the obstruction lesion, seem more dangerous and may well lead to a greater chance of pneumothorax because of trapped gases under high pressure. Thus the Venturi system seems more suitable.

Insufflation techniques are employed by allowing the patient to breathe spontaneously and then delivering anesthetic agents through a catheter in the pharynx or a device attached to the laryngoscope. This presents the hazard of filling the operative surroundings with anesthetic gases that tend to contaminate the surgeon and operating personnel. This, therefore, would seem a less desirable technique.

If Venturi ventilation is employed, the patient is reintubated at the completion of the procedure and the tube is left in place until the patient is awake and in full control of laryngeal reflexes.

The stainless steel tube of Norton,[6] which was introduced in 1978, does remove the danger of fire, but continues to give the problem of obstruction

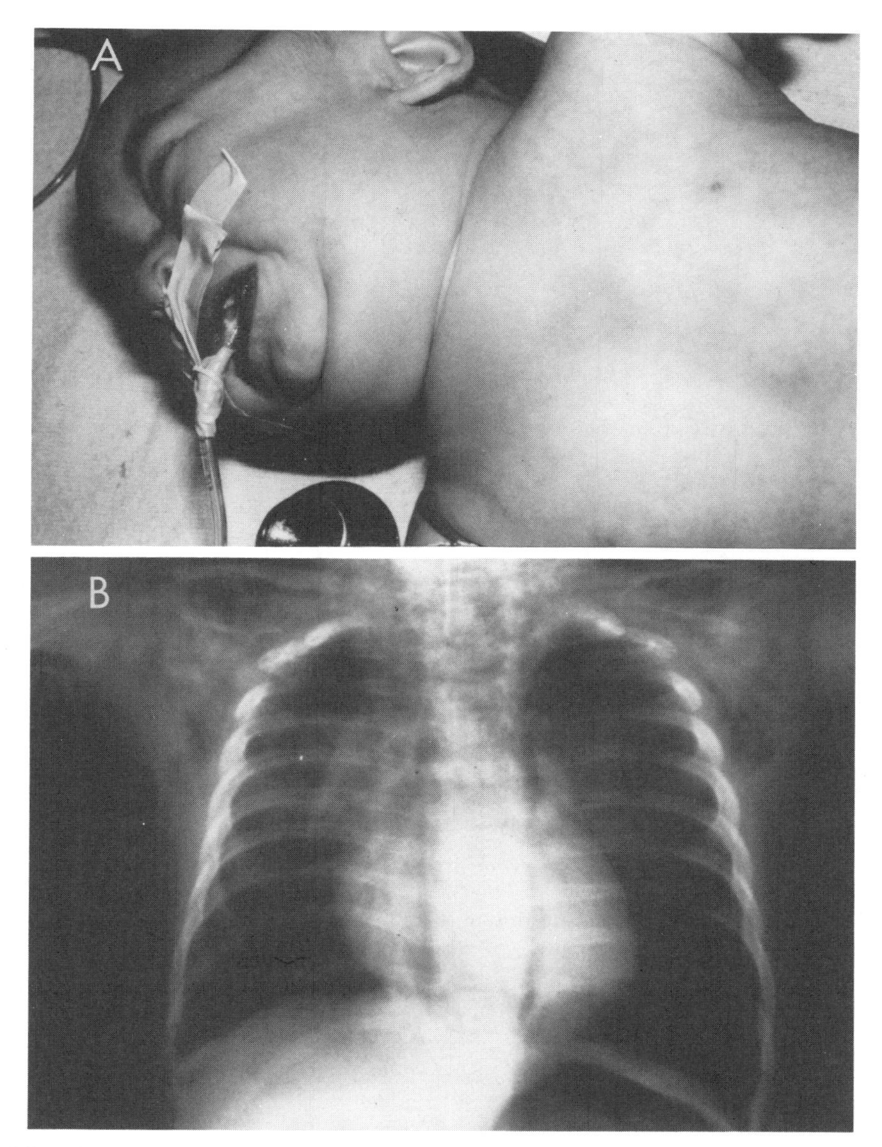

Fig 10–4. **A,** severe subcutaneous emphysema in infant after bilateral pneumothorax secondary to Venturi jet injection ventilation. **B,** chest x-ray showing pneumothorax of same patient.

of the larynx by a tube, and therefore, seems less desirable in pediatrics than in adult laser surgery.

If an endotracheal tube fire should occur, the tube must be immediately removed and the patient ventilated through a mask. Sufficient muscle relaxants should be given to prevent laryngospasm and the airway should be secured. The surgeon must fully examine the entire respiratory tract to determine the extent of injury from the fire. Tracheotomy may be necessary in cases of extensive injury and in such cases antibiotics and corticosteroids should be given.

LASER INSTRUMENT COMPLICATIONS

Any complication that may be attributable to nonlaser microlaryngeal surgery or bronchoscopy may occur during laser surgery. This includes damaged teeth, tongue edema, laryngeal edema, and cervical spine injury. Therefore, the same precautions must be exercised as would be done during any microsurgical procedure.

Partial malalignment of the laser system mirrors may result in energy loss, and thus, a diffuse, poorly focused beam. This may lead to uneven depths of penetration, and thus, an undesirable result. The laser must be carefully checked and tested before the procedure begins to assure that this is not happening.

Heat injury due to malalignment of the laser bronchoscope is always a possibility. If care is not taken to continuously monitor the external temperature of the bronchoscope, then an unsuspected burn to the skin or mucosal surfaces may take place. This, therefore, requires diligent and meticulous attention by the surgeon. It is essential that proper alignment of the bronchoscope and laser be established prior to each procedure.

It is also necessary to maintain constant vigilance during laser bronchoscopy to assure that small fragments of tissue do not become detached and impacted distal to the area of resection. It is usually best to pass the bronchoscope distal to the lesion to be removed to gain airway control, and then move proximally with the resection to maintain patency of the airway.

The patient's face should be completely protected from inadvertent laser injury by the use of moistened eye pads and either moistened towels or gauze sponges (Fig 10–5). These must be kept continuously wet, and will provide some degree of protection from an inadvertent laser burst. It is important that the assistant control the activation of the laser system any time the surgeon stops lasering. This may be necessary several times during the case, but ensures that an inadvertent injury to either the patient or surrounding personnel will not occur. The surgeon and OR personnel should

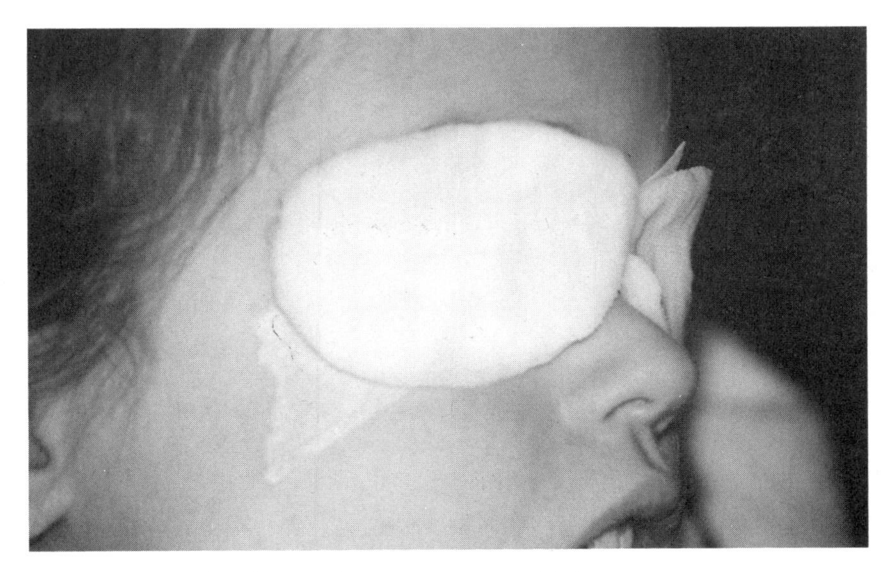

Fig 10–5. Moist sponges utilized to protect eyes.

take precautions to protect their eyes, as this represents the greatest hazard to those involved in the surgical procedure. The use of corrective lenses or goggles is strongly recommended.

SUMMARY

The CO_2 laser has proven to be an extremely effective and useful tool in pediatrics. It has allowed the transoral endoscopic correction of several problems that formerly required open procedures. Its use is not without complication, however, and requires extreme diligence on the part of the surgeon and OR personnel to ensure that an unfortunate incident does not occur during its usage. Meticulous attention to detail and appropriate training are absolutely essential to keep the possibility of complication at the most minimal level.

REFERENCES

1. Strong M.S., Jako G.J.: Laser surgery in the larynx. *Ann. Otol. Rhinol. Laryngol.* 81:791–798, 1972.
2. Burgess G.E., LeJeune F.E.: Endotracheal tube ignition during laser surgery of the larynx. *Arch. Otolaryngol.* 105:561–562, 1979.

3. Meyers A.: Complications of CO_2 laser surgery of the larynx. *Ann. Otol. Rhinol. Laryngol.* 90:132–134, 1981.
4. Healy G.B., Strong M.S., Shapshay S., et al.: Complications of CO_2 laser surgery of the aerodigestive tract: Experience of 4416 cases. *Otolaryngol. Head Neck Surg.* 92:13–18, 1984.
5. Woo P., Eurenius S.: The dynamics of Venturi jet ventilation through the operating laryngoscope. *Ann. Otol. Rhinol. Laryngol.* 91:615–621, 1982.
6. Norton M.L., DeVos P.: New endotracheal tube for laser surgery of the larynx. *Ann. Otol. Rhinol. Laryngol.* 87:554–557, 1978.

11 Nursing Aspects in Operative Laser Surgery

Brenda J. McKonly, R.N., M.S.

Carol A. Richard, R.N.

The use of lasers in surgery has grown rapidly during the past decade. Most medical centers have at least one laser and often several types. The surgical benefits of lasers are being realized in community hospitals as well. With this surge in the use of these instruments comes an increase in nursing's responsibility to understand the principles of laser surgery, the laser unit, and the safety measures necessary to assure safe patient care.

In this chapter the authors will review nursing's administrative responsibilities during and after the purchasing decision, the educational requirements, personnel and patient safety measures, room preparation, and the nursing preventive management of potential complications.

ADMINISTRATIVE MEASURES

Decision to Buy

The purchase of a laser unit is critical to any hospital organization. Operating room managers must be involved in the laser purchasing decisions. They should be involved from the outset, since they will have valuable input in the determination of which unit to purchase. Operating room managers can assist by completing an assessment of laser users to determine the present and potential laser needs.

This assessment should be systematic. A review of statistics will indicate the actual number of potential laser procedures. This statistical review will also indicate a suggested case mix. Some specialities may require a certain type of laser unit. Higher wattage capabilities may be required by other specialties. This review can help identify which type of laser (CO_2, argon, or Nd:YAG) would be the best investment.

Another component of the assessment should include a survey of all surgeons to determine which ones plan to use the laser and for which procedures. It might be important to discuss with the potential users just how strong their commitment is to using this instrument. A comparison of the surgeon's predicted use with the actual figures from the previous year would give the OR manager an estimate of the potential use.

Another aspect of predicting the potential use is an analysis of area hospitals. Inquiries should be made regarding the type of units owned, the type of procedures being done, the number of procedures being done, and the specialties using the laser. If a group of surgeons share facilities, it is of the utmost importance that this investigation is thorough. Duplicating an expensive unit for a relatively small patient population could be quite costly.

Once the usage is estimated, the emphasis must be focused on predicting the future needs. With the critical advances being made today, care must be taken to reduce the possibility of the unit chosen becoming outdated in a short time span. Current financial constraints place a heavy emphasis on using money wisely.

Financial consideration is probably the most important facet of the purchasing decision. Along with the cost of the basic unit, monies budgeted must include those attachments needed for various specialties, any special plumbing or wiring needed for installation, a plume evacuation system, a service contract, and educational programs for medical and nursing staffs. The ongoing expense of gas tanks and regulators must be evaluated when planning operational costs. Many agencies establish an additional charge for laser use during surgical procedures. According to Pfister and Kneedler,[1] a good rule of thumb is, "If the laser would be used for fifteen procedures per month, you can justify the purchase of a $100,000 laser."[1] Many creative options exist for financing a laser, such as leasing, buying outright, fund-raising drives, or special charge per usage arrangements. All options should be explored simultaneously while evaluating the many types available on the market today.

All of the previous factors should be evaluated prior to the organization's decision to purchase a laser. What one wants to accomplish is to purchase the best unit for the money and needs. After the purchase decision has been made, the hospital must then prepare for the safe use of the unit.

Laser Safety Program

With the purchase of a surgical laser comes the need to assure its proper use in the delivery of safe patient care. Administrative responsibilities require that a plan be developed to implement a laser safety program based on the organization's unique needs. The plan should include requirements for the introduction of all new equipment and also those principles and standards of laser safety.

As with all new electrical equipment being introduced into the system, lasers must be evaluated and examined by the biomedical engineering department. When this approval is obtained, the laser may be available for appropriate patient use. The biomedical engineers may be called on for routine maintenance of the laser unit, such as safety checks, repair of electrical cords, and changing fuses. However, any specific maintenance beyond the routine must be done by specialized company representatives. All safety committees should include a member of the biomedical engineering department.

The development of a laser safety committee that assumes accountability for all aspects of safe laser use is strongly recommended. The committee responsibilities should include the review and adherence of standards; writing, reviewing, revising, and approving policies and procedures; and the establishment of the credentialing requirements. The committee should continue to evaluate the ongoing laser needs. The committee may be a new committee formed or a subcommittee of the already established OR committee. Suggested membership might be the following:

Medical staff representative from each specialty
Anesthesia staff representative
OR director
OR head nurses responsible for specialties planning to use the laser
Nursing representatives from other areas where the laser might be used, for example, ambulatory clinics
Biomedical engineer
Representative from administration
The laser coordinator.

Adherence to the guidelines and standards set by several bodies is the duty of this committee. Some examples of these bodies are American National Standards Institute, Inc., Joint Commission on Accreditation of Hospitals, Occupational Safety and Health Administration, FDA (particularly the Medical Device Amendments), and your state regulators.

Using standards, individual committees can develop their own policies and procedures that serve as guidelines to staff and employees for the safe use of the laser. The following are suggested areas to be addressed by the committee:

Function of the laser committee
Responsibility of the laser team (physicians, nurses, and coordinator)
Requirements of medical staff for credentialing

Requirements of other personnel for credentialing
Patient safety precautions
Personnel safety precautions
Fire prevention protocols
Preventative maintenance
Instrumentation use
Plume evacuation guidelines
Patient consent forms
Accident reporting mechanism
Proper documentation of all laser procedures
Charge procedure.

The committee should address the above listed policies and procedures but, of course, not be limited to them.

The credentialing requirements are established to protect the patient and staff during laser surgery. A set of prescribed requirements substantiates the surgeon's qualifications to perform laser surgery. The credentialing process must include proof that the requesting surgeon has completed a recognized course in laser surgery with "hands-on experience." These courses are being offered more frequently at various locations. Next, the requesting surgeon must demonstrate knowledge of the laser unit to the designated surgeon preceptor in laser. And third, the requesting surgeon must be able to demonstrate expertise in laser surgery. This is usually accomplished by working with a designated surgeon preceptor for a predetermined number of times. It is after successful completion of these three steps that the preceptor will recommend to the committee that the requesting surgeon be granted laser surgery privileges. All surgeons should be notified in writing of their approval with copies forwarded to the chief of surgery and the OR director. All operating privileges must be maintained permanently in the OR director's office. To ease the scheduling process, notification of the surgeon's privilege must be communicated to the scheduling coordinator as soon as possible.

Scheduling

As the use of lasers increases, scheduling will become more complex. The assurance of the unit's availability becomes crucial. Some units are portable and can be transported safely to the needed room. Others are stationary, so the room designed for the laser hookup must be able to easily accommodate the specialties that plan to use that laser. With more and more surgeons using the laser in the future, simultaneous bookings can become a problem if not guarded against by an astute scheduling coordinator. If a computer is used, double booking of equipment can be prevented by appropriate programming. If a unit is out for repair, scheduling must be alerted immediately so already scheduled procedures can be accommodated or surgeons notified of potential lack of equipment.

In addition to availability and location issues, scheduling policies must allot time for any accessory equipment to be ready for the scheduled procedure. This may be the various endoscopy or eye equipment used with the Nd:YAG laser or the appropriate sizes of the stapes protheses to be used with the argon laser. An allowance of time must be given for adequate reprocessing of lenses and fiberoptic cables.

Scheduling requires the coordination of many departments to assure the safest care for patients. Planning ahead through established scheduling policies may help to reduce conflicts and potential risks.

Nursing Education

To ensure the success of a laser program, it is necessary to provide introductory and ongoing training of OR personnel. Emphasis is placed on the day-to-day operation of the laser and of new developments with its widespread use.

When planning a laser-orientation program for the department the OR manager or instructor must consider the needs of the staff based on their individual roles and the type of laser to be used in surgery.

The entire OR staff including ancillary personnel should attend the laser inservice program. In some cases, orderlies may be required to assist the nurse in transporting a laser unit. A basic understanding of the component will eliminate the possibility of bumping or jarring the system. Such movement will cause a misalignment of the internal mirrors that are used to direct the laser beam of the CO_2 laser.

In addition to alleviating any fears associated with the new device, the content of the program should include laser physics, mechanics of lasers, types of lasers, and specific characteristics of the commonly used surgical units, safety factors, and measures to be taken in the event of an emergency.

Physicians should be encouraged to participate in the program, demonstrating the clinical applications of lasers as related to their specialty, and the prospects of new developments as lasers are further explored.

Nursing responsibilities during laser surgery should be clearly defined to provide optimal patient care and to adequately assist the surgeon during the procedure.

There are several resources available to assist the manager in implementing the teaching process. Laser manufacturers can provide literature as well as inservice programs on the use of the laser equipment. This information is usually technical in nature and often fails to incorporate aspects of patient care and nursing responsibilities.

Recent medical and nursing journals are considered the current source of laser information as related to surgical specialties. These publications define the nursing role during surgical laser intervention and assist in establishing standards necessary to provide optimal patient care.

The OR manager may employ the services of a nurse consultant to introduce the concept of laser surgery at the time of installation of a laser system. The consultant may present an inservice program or a one-day workshop.[1] There are increasing numbers of surgical laser workshops and seminars available for the staff to attend that will provide basic nursing education.

Although a laser introduction program is mandatory for all staff members, it is said that the hands-on experience gained is invaluable. The OR manager should select a registered nurse to serve as a laser coordinator. This individual need not have had previous laser experience, however, he or she should have an interest in laser surgery. It is imperative that this individual complete a recognized laser course and work closely with the laser consultant during the initial planning stages as well as when the first laser procedures are performed.[1]

The laser coordinator and a select group of nursing personnel should participate in an intensive training program. The selection of nurses is based on the type of laser used and the procedures to be performed. If a laser is purchased for a specific surgical specialty, the manager may wish to provide in-depth knowledge to nurses who have expertise in this area.[1] These nurses will eventually assume the role of preceptors and will assist in the education of other staff members as they are assigned to that procedure or specialty.

This intense training program may be provided by the nurse-consultant. Specific characteristics of the laser and its interaction on tissue should be explained. The nurse's role in preparing the laser for surgical application needs to be demonstrated.

Knowledge is gained through experience. Return demonstrations of laser setup and applied safety measures reinforce basic principles of laser technology.

The laser coordinator must be a member of the Laser Safety Committee. The committee participates in the development of written policies and procedures that will define the scope of nursing responsibilities in laser surgery. As new developments occur, the committee shall review and evaluate the policies and revise them accordingly. The responsibility of the laser coordinator is to keep the staff informed of any changes and assist them in achieving good standards of care.

An operating manual should be provided and located on each laser system within the department. It will serve as a resource for nursing personnel and should be reviewed prior to the start of a laser procedure. In addition to general product information, including system setup, it should contain a laser safety checklist. Designed to serve as a guide for providing continuity of patient care, this checklist will enable nurses to enforce specific procedures as established by the Laser Safety Committee. The last section of this manual may serve as a procedure log. Here, pertinent information about the patient and procedure are recorded.

Continuing educational programs must be provided on a yearly basis. Effective education of personnel in the safe and knowledgeable use of the laser tool will aid in prevention of laser-related accidents. The purpose of ongoing training is to allow the staff to review basic laser concepts, reinforce safety measures to be employed, and maintain competence in the practical use and application of laser equipment. Finally, continuing education programs augment knowledge pertinent to new developments in patient care.

LASER SAFETY

Along with the laser's unique ability to cut and coagulate tissues is the inherent danger to potentially injure healthy tissue. Strict adherence to safety rules will prevent accidents and injury.

There are two major dangers to patients and personnel working with the laser. First, the laser beam may either directly or by reflection strike an unprotected area of the patient or staff member. Secondly, the beam may strike an unprotected endotracheal tube, puncturing it, mixing with oxygen, and causing it to ignite.[2]

Because of the potential dangers to patients and personnel, the laser should be used in a restricted area. Operating rooms provide this restriction, which helps to reduce the traffic to only those individuals necessary for patient care. Another protective measure is the posting of the standard red sun-burst signs on all entrances to the room where the laser unit is being used. All personnel should know the minimal safety measures of protective eyewear and traffic reduction. Some facilities have a system set up whereby a warning light outside and above the door is illuminated when the laser unit is activated by the foot switch. This provides clear communication to all individuals who may be considering entrance into the laser room.

All laser types are hazardous to unprotected eyes. The CO_2 laser is primarily dangerous to the cornea; the argon laser is primarily dangerous to the retina, and the Nd:YAG laser beam is intense at its focal point and creates shocks posterior to the lens. Its damage can be deep and penetrating. Because of the potential damage to eyes, all personnel must wear protective eyewear. If patients undergo procedures under local anesthetics, they too must wear the eyeglasses. The glasses should have sides to provide peripheral protection. Corrective eyeglasses may also be worn, but afford protection for only the CO_2 laser. Contact lenses do not provide adequate protection. If the laser is attached to a microscope, the surgeon does not need protective eyewear in addition to binocular microscope lenses.

Clear glasses are worn when the CO_2 laser is being used. Orange to red-tinted glasses are worn when the argon laser is being used, because they absorb the impact of the blue-green beam. Faint blue or green-tinted glasses are worn when the Nd:YAG is being used. If an endoscope is being used with the Nd:YAG, the eyepiece must be fitted to protect the operator.

When using the CO_2 laser for head and neck procedures, the patient's eyes and surrounding skin must be protected. The most effective method is with moist gauze or cotton over the eyes. The lips and nose should be covered with moist gauze or towels. It is important to keep all combustibles moist throughout the entire procedure, because the CO_2 beam is absorbed by water.

The second major danger is fire in the airway. This is the most serious complication in laser surgery, particularly laryngeal surgery. Several safety measures must be taken to prevent this complication (see chapters 3 and 5).

Safety measures to reduce the major danger of fires are extremely important. They must be reviewed constantly with all involved personnel. Other risks with the laser are related to electrical hazards and gas tank precautions. As with all electrical equipment, biomedical engineering must be notified immediately if any problem arises. The unit should not be used if there are frayed cords. Routine maintenance checks should be done as a preventive measure. Storage, handling, and the use of gas tanks with the lasers need to be handled in accordance with regulations already being followed for all other gas tanks in all ORs.

All safety measures must be stressed with personnel working with the laser. Taking care to adhere to these measures can reduce potential risks to all patients and personnel.

NURSING CARE

The laser coordinator will play an active role in the perioperative care of the patient. As experience is gained, standard perioperative protocols should be developed to provide continuity of care. The protocols should be evaluated and revised as needed to provide improved standards as advances are made in the field of laser surgery.

Preoperative Preparation

The laser coordinator and/or designated team member interviews the patient prior to surgery and participates in the development of a care plan specific to the surgical procedure and patient's needs.

Whether the surgery is on an inpatient or ambulatory basis, it is advantageous for the nurse to interview the patient and possibly family members as well. Because of attention given to lasers by the media, the patient may be extremely apprehensive and misinformed. Some laser treatments are in the experimental stages and until long-term results are available, can not be considered a cure-all for all diseases. For example, laser treatment for the patient with diabetic retinopathy will not restore sight, it merely prevents further loss of vision.

Patients need to know basic information and why it has been selected as the treatment of choice for their particular disorder. It is important for nursing to have acquired specific laser information, including unique properties, physics, and characteristics of the commonly used lasers. The nurses will reinforce information received from the patient's physician, and clarify misconceptions the patient may have regarding surgery. Any unresolved issues should be referred back to the physician.

Similar to preoperative interviews completed on all surgical patients, the nurse gathers the appropriate information from the patient and his or her records, including laboratory test results. Past and present physical history information is collected, and a physical assessment is made to complete the care plan. A brief review of the day's events will be explained to the patient, and any further questions will be answered.

In summary, the preoperative interview will establish the rapport needed to alleviate fears, provide patient education, and prepare the patient for surgery.

Intraoperative Nursing Responsibilities

On arrival to the OR or preoperative holding area, the patient is greeted by the secretary or nurse-in-charge and the admission process is initiated. A systematic review of the preoperative check-list is followed by gathering other admission data including laboratory test results. The surgical consent form is reviewed and verified for its accuracy.

To date the Nd:YAG laser is considered an investigational device by the FDA. The FDA requires a consent form to specify the laser being used and to list its potential complications. Such complications include the following:

Massive bleeding
Perforation
Gas embolization
Dissemination of viable cells
Distention
Fever, sepsis, and pain
Danger of combustion and fire
Possible death due to massive bleeding, organ perforation, and combustion.

The consent form should also include a statement giving the right of the FDA and laser manufacturer to examine records.[1]

Nursing should attempt to alleviate patients' fears by answering any questions they may have. It is important to provide emotional support and help to reduce the patient's anxiety.

Prior to the arrival of the patient to the OR, the laser and its accessories should be assembled. Selected instruments are sterilized and made ready for the procedure. The laser key is secured.

Laser warning signs are posted on the doors leading into the OR. Appropriate eye protection is provided for all personnel assigned to the case.

Instruments and accessories for laser surgery are determined by the type of laser used and the procedure to be performed.

Instruments used near the laser beam must be surface treated as reflection of the beam off shiny instrument surfaces is a primary hazard (Fig 11–1). Ebonizing chemically changes the surface of stainless steel by an electromagnetic process. The surface will wear away eventually and the process must be repeated. Black nickel plating is the process of applying nickel to the stainless steel surface. It is a durable process and will withstand repeated steam sterilizations. Black chroming is a process where a high grade of black chromium is applied to a dispersive surface. Mirrors are often used to reflect the laser beam into an area unable to be reached by direct beam. The surgeon must exercise caution to avoid hitting an undesired target. Microlaryngeal surgery with the use of the CO_2 laser will require surface-treated laryngoscopes, suction tips, retractors, and mirrors. Pfister and Kneedler[1] discourage the use of standard glass laryngeal mirrors, stating they have a tendency to pit. Crystals will begin to flake off after the mirror has been struck with the laser beam several times.[1]

The free-hand attachment used in CO_2 laser surgery consists of a metal handpiece connecting to a lens, which in turn is attached to the end of the

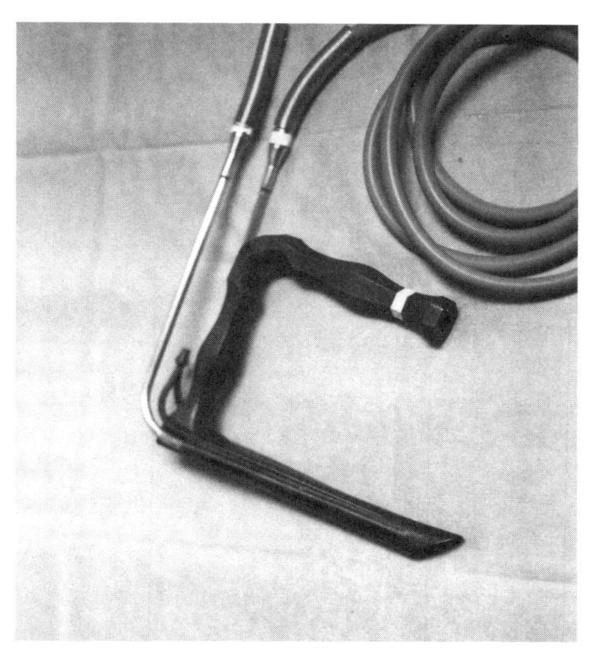

Fig 11–1. Laryngoscope, ebonized to reduce the laser beam reflection.

articulating arm. The surgeon holds the handpiece like a pencil and directs the beam to the affected tissue. The metal handpiece can be steam sterilized prior to use. Because it is a prism, the lens will not withstand steam sterilization (Fig 11–2). Cooling gases blow across the lens of many CO_2 laser units and may contribute to the introduction of microorganisms into the wound.[1] Therefore, it is recommended that a lens be cleaned with at least a 95% alcohol solution after each use.[1]

Since the free-hand and articulating arm is positioned directly over the sterile field, it is necessary to drape it with a transparent disposable sterile drape. Manufacturers have designed numerous sterile drapes that will assist in maintaining a sterile field and enable the surgeon to visualize the joints in the articulating arm (Fig 11–3). For clean procedures, sterilized handpieces are placed on the laser without draping the laser arm.

In laryngeal surgery, the lens is part of the microscope adaptor. This adaptor allows the laser to be coupled with the microscope and enables the laser beam to be directed through a laryngoscope or bronchoscope (Fig 11–4).

Additional accessories requested for microlaryngeal surgery may include extra viewing devices, video tape equipment, and camera attachments.

Many ORs have developed floor plans to assist personnel in setting up

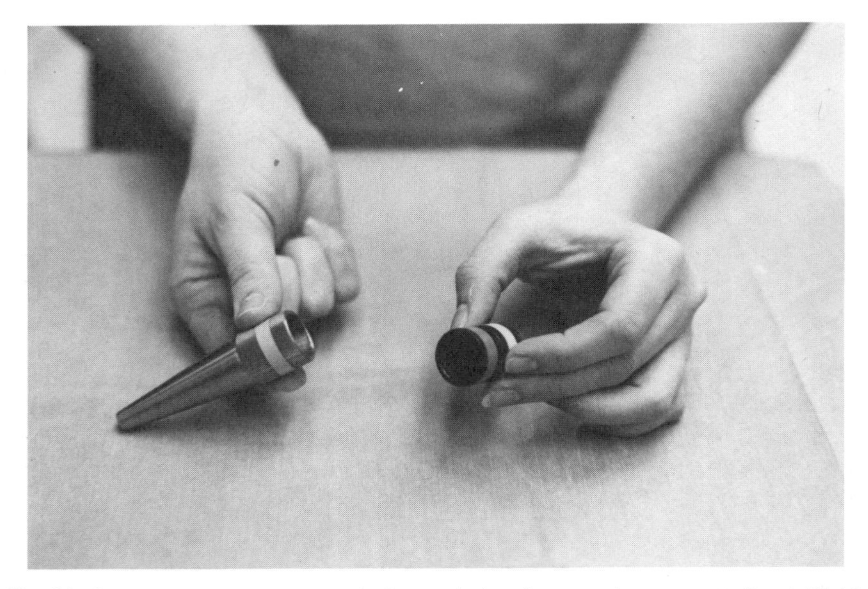

Fig 11–2. Hand-held attachment. **Left,** metal, therefore may be steam sterilized. **Right,** lens, therefore will not withstand steam sterilization.

necessary equipment. These plans will reduce the possibility of potential complications associated with overcrowding of equipment.[1]

The laser should be checked for proper functioning. Most CO_2 lasers have an internal cooling mechanism and do not need special external hookups. Some CO_2 lasers have external gas cylinders that must be checked before and during the procedure.

The argon and Nd:YAG laser systems have external cooling mechanisms. The argon laser must be connected to an outside water source for a period of time before and after its use. This will allow cooling of the laser tube. Proper water levels must be maintained to aid in cooling the system. Some argon lasers are air cooled and must be checked for proper fan function. Air filters used in this system must be changed as needed.

When assembling and testing the laser, the nurse should follow the guidelines distributed by the manufacturers and the hospital protocol. Test firing on a wet tongue blade will confirm proper alignment of the aiming beam.[1]

The plume and odors generated by the vaporization of tissue during laser surgery may be vented by means of a smoke evacuator. The filter contained in the evacuation system, if used, must be checked and replaced as necessary.

Positoning

During laryngoscopy surgery, the patient is supine with a degree of neck hyperextension in order to introduce the laryngoscope and attach the suspension equipment. The surgeon will work from the head of the table while the anesthesiologist maintains adequate ventilation at the patient's side.

The laser and instrument table should be positioned to one side of the surgeon and the microscope will enter from the opposite side (Fig 11–5).

Positioning for free-hand CO_2 laser and argon laser surgery is dependent on the location of the area to be treated. Patients are usually supine, with the affected area exposed. Eye protection is secured as the patient is positioned for surgery. Awake patients will wear the same glasses as the OR personnel.

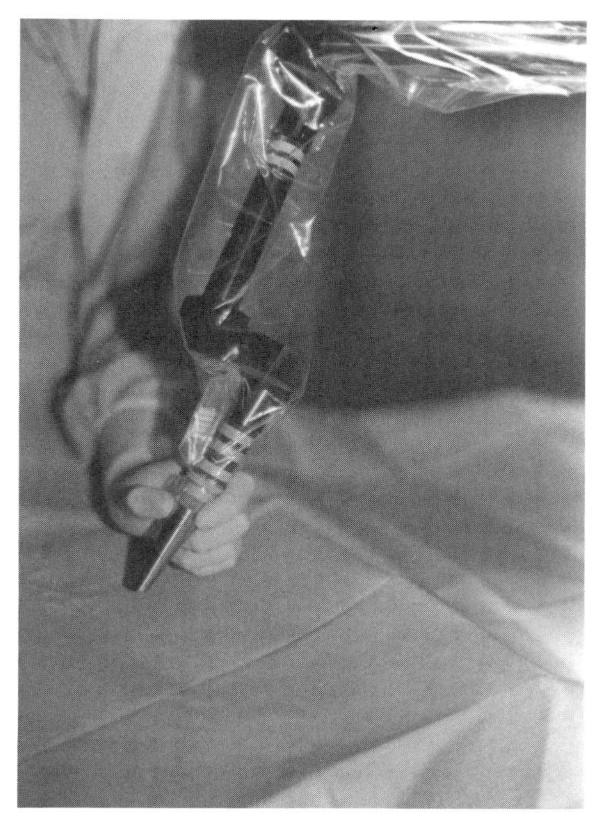

Fig 11–3. Draping the articulating arm of the laser.

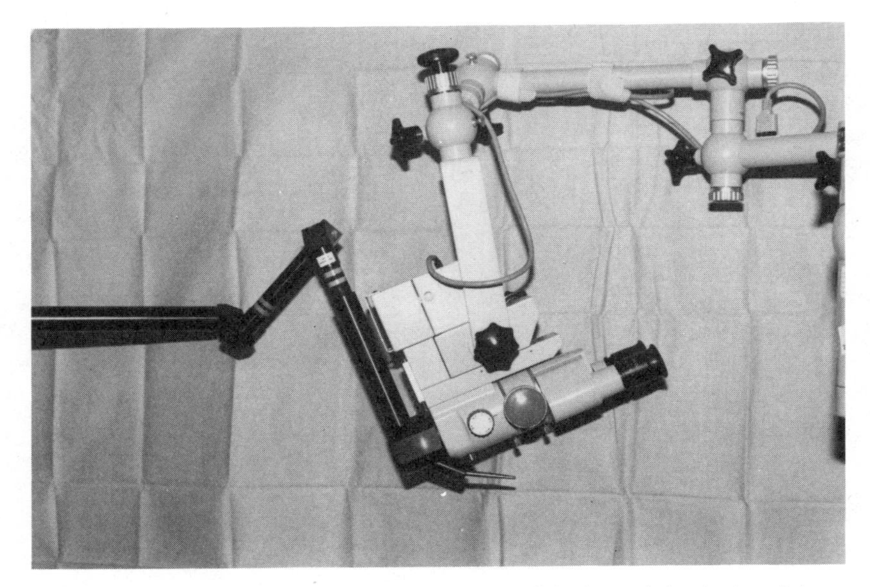

Fig 11–4. Microscope adaptor. Manipulation of the beam is by the joy stick.

Prepping and Draping the Patient

Patients undergoing CO_2 laser surgery must be prepared with a nonflammable solution. Because it is a combustible agent, alcohol is contraindicated as a prepping solution.

Draping is similar as for conventional surgery. Drapes surrounding the operative site must be protected with moistened sponges or towels to prevent a fire when using the CO_2 laser.[1] To avoid moisture contamination, the use of impervious draping material is recommended.

In laryngeal surgery, the patient's teeth are protected with plastic tooth guards to prevent chipping. Moistened sponges and eye pads are placed over the eyes, lips, and tongue. Wet cottonoids are placed around the wrapped endotracheal tube. The scrub nurse must closely observe the area surrounding the operative site. Moistened sponge and cottonoids must be continuously saturated with saline.[1]

To prevent accidental discharge, the laser should be in a standby mode when not in use. Do not leave a laser while in use. Select a mode and adjust wattage as requested by the surgeon.

Depending on the type of laser system in use, vacuum pressure dials and gas tanks should be checked periodically.

Intraoperative nursing notes should include patient position and any protective activities performed. These notes should also include the type of laser used, the length of time the laser was used, and the power and exposure times.[1]

In the logbook accompanying the laser, the nurse records the patient name, date, type of surgery, the laser setting, and time of exposure. Complications must be reported to the Laser Safety Committee and follow-up documentation will be necessary.

The circulating nurses must monitor the activity in the room by enforcing safety regulations and acting as the patient advocate. They will enforce wearing the appropriate eye protection and control traffic in and out of the room during the laser procedure.

Endotracheal Tube Fire

A fire in the airway is the most serious complication of laser surgery. Endotracheal fires require immediate action by the surgical team. A fire pro-

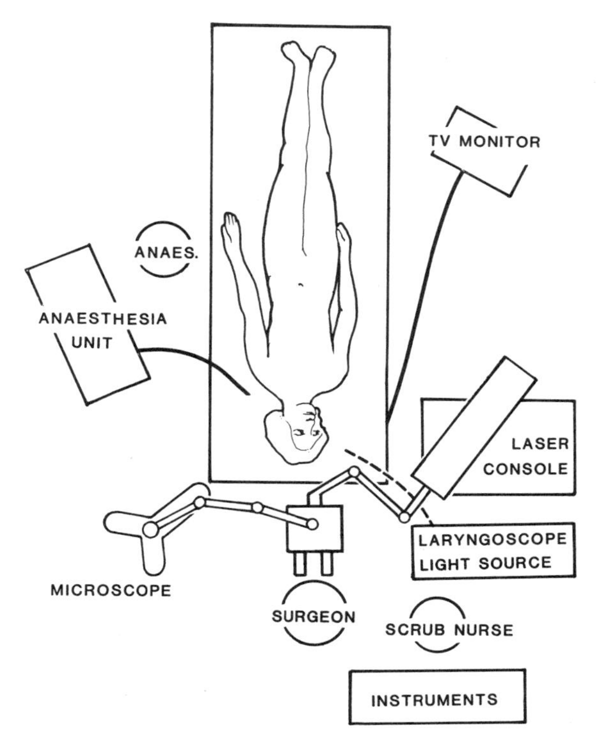

Fig 11–5. Typical laser laryngoscope organization in OR. Equipment is placed to prevent clutter.

cedure should be established by the Laser Safety Committee and reviewed by the staff prior to the start of the case. The following equipment must be readily available:

Oral airway
Anesthesia mask
Small cuffed or uncuffed endotracheal tube
Rigid ventilating bronchoscope
Rod telescope
Large foreign-body forceps
Flexible fiberoptic bronchoscope
Laryngoscope
Tracheotomy tray
Low-pressure cuffed tracheotomy tube

A fire protocol has been developed by Schramm[3]. He distinguishes between primary and secondary emergency action following an endotracheal tube fire. Primary care includes the simultaneous cessation of ventilation, brief discontinuance of oxygenation, and removal of the endotracheal tube. The removal of the burning endotracheal tube is the prime consideration. Oxygen itself will not burn and continued oxygenation of the patient is mandatory.

Secondary emergency care consists of reintubation using a smaller tube or ventilating bronchoscope. Rigid and flexible bronchoscopies are performed to remove foreign bodies and carbon debris, to lavage the trachea and distal airways and evaluate the tracheobronchial tree. Fragmented mucosa is removed during direct laryngoscopy and pharyngoscopy. If necessary, a tracheotomy may be performed.

By following the safety policies established by the Laser Safety Committee, those who play an active role in laser surgery will aid in fire prevention.

POSTOPERATIVE CONSIDERATIONS

Postanesthesia nurses should be included in the laser-orientation program. They must know the physiological responses and possible complications following laser surgery and how to respond to them. Protocols and procedures must be established as a guide in order to meet the needs of the patient following their specific procedure.[1]

Postoperative care after laser surgery is similar to the care given to patients following surgery using conventional methods. A proper airway must be maintained and the cardiovascular status monitored. The operative site should be checked for bleeding and pain medication administered as needed for any discomfort.

Laser vaporization of tissue will cause the surgical area to dry out. Therefore, postanesthesia care for the patient having laryngeal surgery may include the application of humidified oxygen for lubrication of the vocal cords. Some patients are prone to nausea and vomiting following general anesthesia. Since vomiting will interfere with the crusting of vaporized cells in the throat, it is important to alleviate these symptoms.[1] If suctioning is required, it should be done lightly to avoid irritating the laser-treated area.

Patients may be on voice rest for 24 to 48 hours and may experience hoarseness for several weeks following their treatment. The first meal will often consist of a liquid diet. A soft diet may be ordered for the second meal and subsequent nourishment is determined by patient's tolerance and physician's preference. Written postprocedure instructions are based on individual patient needs. A copy of the instructions shall be given to the patient on discharge. Time is provided to answer any questions the patient may have about the surgery and to clarify the postoperative instructions. It should be emphasized that due to the minimal damage to surrounding tissue during laser surgery, there is a reduction in the amount of postoperative pain and edema. There is also a minimal tendency to scar formation. Patients having facial laser surgery may forget they have had a treatment and accidentally scratch or rub the area. This can result in delayed healing and may cause bleeding and scarring.

Following a laser treatment, the pigmentation process may be affected. Patients should avoid exposure to sunlight for up to a year. The use of sunblocking agents and protective clothing may be necessary during this time.[1]

Due to a high anxiety level preoperatively, the patient may experience exhaustion following surgery. The nurse should allow a sufficient recouperating period prior to initiating discharge instructions.

Many ambulatory centers will contact the patients after discharge from the hospital to check on their progress and reinforce the physician's instructions.

SUMMARY

Laser surgery offers unique advantages to patients. Their use will become far greater in the future. Health care agencies have a responsibility to acquire the type of laser that best meets the needs of their community's patient population. The OR managers must take an active role in the purchasing decision, the establishment of a safe laser program, the initial and ongoing education of all personnel, and the assurance of safe nursing practice during the perioperative phase of the surgical experience. The technological advances yet to come in the laser surgical field shall prove to be exciting for nursing.

REFERENCES

1. Pfister J., Kneedler J.A.: *A Guide to Lasers in the O.R.* Aurora, Ill., Education Design/Editorial Consultants, 1983.
2. Carruth A.L., Wainwright A.C.: The carbon dioxide laser: Safety aspects. *J. Laryngol. Otol.* 94:411–417, 1980.
3. Schramm V.L. Jr., Mattox D.E., Stool S.E.: Acute management of laser ignited intratracheal explosion. *Laryngoscope* 91:1417–1426, 1981.

BIBLIOGRAPHY

1. Hirshman C.A., Smith J.L.: Indirect ignition of the endotracheal tube during carbon dioxide laser surgery. *Arch. Otolaryngol.* 106:636–641, 1980.
2. Meyers A.D.: Complications of CO_2 laser surgery of the larynx. *Ann. Otol.* 90:132–134, 1981.
3. Meyers A.D., Fay M.F.: The laser as a surgical tool. *Today's O.R. Nurse* 1:14–21, 1979.
4. Fried M.P.: Complications of CO_2 laser surgery of the larynx. *Laryngoscope* 93:275–278, 1983.
5. Carrell B.L.: Laser treatment of laryngeal polyps. *AORN J.* 38:232–236, 1983.
6. Steven D.L.: Use of the carbon dioxide laser in your operating room. *J. Operating Room Research Institute* 2:7–11, 1982.
7. Steffers V.: Safety checklist documents responsibilities of the laser nurse. *Clin. Laser Month.* 2:55, 1984.
8. Xanar, Inc.: *Guidelines for Establishing a Hospital Laser Program.* Colorado Springs, CO, 1983.
9. Gray F.N.: CO_2 Lasers—Everything you wanted to know about lasers . . . and more! *Today's O.R. Nurse* 6:14–21, 1984.

12

Medical Lasers and the Law

Martin L. Norton, M.D., J.D.

Edward V. Norton, J.D.

"There are many lights in light."
Talmud, Berachot 52 b.

Lasers present legal problems similar to other medical devices in the market place. For the physician-practitioner, there are issues related to negligence law. For the manufacturer and distributor there are the dual problems of products liability and regulatory laws.[1]

This presentation will discuss some of the more pertinent aspects under the three categories of negligence, regulatory laws, and products' liability. The physician-reader will note, and hopefully be alerted to the fact that he or she is touched directly or indirectly by all three considerations. This discussion is intended to inform, but will not be a primer on all the nuances of the law. We trust it will contribute to understanding and thus ease the way for future developments in laser medicine. While we may discuss these generically, we must always keep in mind our primary concern—the patient treated with a laser.

NEGLIGENCE

The physician has been made painfully aware of the problems of medical practice through the proliferation of malpractice suits brought in recent years. Issues of informed consent, experimentation, criteria of tort actions, damages, the expert witness, and other aspects will be discussed.

Informed Consent

While consent *per se* would not seem to be a classical tort, most courts currently focus on the materiality[2] of undisclosed information. Here, the plaintiff need only show that this information, if disclosed, would have caused the patient (or a reasonable person) to forego the treatment.[3] Thus, the duty of disclosure is established by judicial interpretation based on the landmark decision of Justice Cardozo,[4] establishing the right of each individual to determine what shall be done to his or her body.

The laser seems to the practitioner to be a simple medium for his or her art. The other chapters of this book may disavow him or her of some of this simplicity. The area most likely to be the nidus for litigation is that of informed consent. We do not stress that aspect of informed consent relating to the specifics of patient injury, but rather refer to (a) the failure of the practitioner to obtain proper training before using the laser instrument; (b) failure to become proficient in the use of a specific instrument and modality; and (c) failure to inform the patient of the level of training and expertise of the laser practitioner.

Appended to this book are the criteria for credentialing in the use of medical lasers promulgated at the University of Michigan Hospitals and as formulated in substance for the American National Standards Institute (ANSI). One notes that they address items (a) and (b) above. Mere observation of laser surgery, or superficial use "under supervision," may be inadequate. Furthermore, each instrument is different, each modality has different characteristics in function, effect, and operational procedures. Expertise with one instrument does not establish competency with another instrument or modality.

The patient is entitled to all information that is material to making an informed judgment on accepting the laser as the instrument of choice. This is particularly important, since in almost all situations there is another surgical alternative, e.g., cold knife, cryotherapy, etc. This concept relates not only to the surgeon, but also to the anesthesiologist in his or her choice of Venturi ventilation in contrast to the various types of endotracheal tubes with their respective inherent risks.

Consent also includes a discussion of the ancillary or supporting systems for laser surgery, including the recognition of the risks of anesthesia and the special techniques of ventilation used during anesthesia for laser surgery of the larynx, trachea, or bronchi. A discussion of Venturi ventilation, with its potential complications, as commented on in the chapter on anesthesia, is definitely in order. It therefore becomes incumbent on both the surgeon and the anesthesiologist to be alerted to and fully aware of the option of the other practitioner in his management of the specific patient. An example of this situation was a case that occurred in Pittsburgh, Pa., where a plastic endotracheal tube was used. The heating of the"protective" foil and underlying tube by the laser caused a fire in the airways to occur. One of the plaintiff's claims was failure of informed consent. While it is incumbent on the anesthesiologist to fully inform his patient, this does not in itself obviate the responsibility of the surgeon who is similarly present. He does have joint and several responsibility, at least, to be aware of what is going on and to be sure that his patient is so informed.

Part of the consent issue is a recognition of the extent to which consent must be obtained. The patient must be advised of the potential plan for the procedure, of the alternatives that are available, and of the potential problems of both or either situation as well as the reasons why there is a choice on the part of the physician for a specific mode of treatment. In a rather unusual decision, one court has gone so far as to say that even totally unacceptable alternatives must be discussed.[5] While this decision does not reflect the general trend, the fact remains that this court did come down with its decision on the basis that "if there is only one choice there is no choice at all." This extreme approach fails to take into account that there was, in fact, an alternative for the patient—namely, not to have the procedure done at all.

On the issue of duty or responsibility, it becomes readily evident that there is an interaction between the surgeon and the patient and the anesthesiologist, that is, teamwork. Thus it is conceivable that the legal principle of joint and several liability would be invoked in this context. Joint and several liability refers to the liability of joint tortfeasors for the same injury to persons or property. It includes those who act together in committing wrongs or whose acts, if independent of each other, unite in causing single injury.[6] Here the plaintiff can institute legal action against either or both of these parties or execute judgment against both.

Human Experimentation vs. Innovative Management

Lasers have caught the imagination of the public and the profession. New applications, however, have not quite kept pace with marketing by the manufacturers. We are, therefore, faced with the question of when an experimental procedure or application becomes first an innovative and ultimately an accepted modality. This author (M.L.N.) addressed the question[7] from the philosophic and sociologic context, coming to the conclusion that the integrity of the physician and the profession is sorely tested. Investigational review boards, human study committees, ethics committees, and the like provide some restraint. However, enthusiasm, ego, and/or the desire to help the patient can work adversely to the patient's interest. Animal experience and practice under supervision is urged before exposing patients to risks that may be, as yet, incompletely understood. Ladimer[8] eloquently expressed the situation as follows:

> The term 'experimentation' must be considered objectively so that it is recognizable as a legitimate scientific endeavor which can be advanced by the recognized research scientist. The legal issue would then become not experimentation versus accepted practice of the art of medicine but an evaluation of the plan and conduct of research in relation to specific fact situations and whether the research was conducted with due regard to the interests of the subject. The law has a duty to comprehend the scope and element of diverse human activity and their places in society if it is to assist in making individual judgment and setting or recognizing general values.

The professionals of the FDA and their advisory panels have assisted with the solution of the dilemma for instrumentation entering the marketplace. This will be discussed below.

Criteria of Tort Actions

A tort action in negligence (malpractice) requires the plaintiff to demonstrate the defendant's (a) duty or responsibility, (b) failure of that duty or responsibility, (c) injury to the patient, and (d) proximate relationship between the failure of duty and that injury.

At this point, we must point out the fact that most legal actions (lawsuits) take place in the lower judicial courts. In fact, many cases are settled out of court. Thus, the predominance of cases will not be found in the literature. Information from the lower courts is primarily anecdotal. Furthermore, because of the relatively short time in which lasers have been in medical use, very few cases have reached the appellate courts, to date, where case reports are documented. Consequently, we discuss legal principles herein on the basis of legal analogy. This is no different than using established principles of physics or chemistry to solve problems or equations in different situations.

Damages—Negligence Actions

The laser surgeon may expose the patient to great risk. This is most manifest in intraluminal surgery such as, but not limited to, the aerodigestive tracts. This is because of proximity to vital structures such as innominate and pulmonary arteries (carinal and primary division bronchial surgery). The physician understands the immediate injury to the patient. However, two areas cause great consternation to physicians. First, there is the claim for damages such as emotional stress, loss of parental or a child's comfort and guidance, loss of consortium, and the like. This concerns the physician because he is usually focused solely on the patient's direct needs.

At law and in practice, we must recognize that the patient's disease and therapy does not exist in a vacuum. The patient as a whole, the interaction of family response, and environmental (sociologic) factors, all determine the functional response of the ill to their disease; and response to therapy, while difficult to quantify in sociologic studies, similarly must be considered.

The second point of contention is the "collateral source rule." This concept asserts[9] that compensation received by the injured party "from a source initially independent of the tortfeasor . . . should not be deducted from the damages which the plaintiff would otherwise collect" from the negligent party. In other words, a tortfeasor may not benefit from the fact that the plaintiff has received money from other sources as a result of defendant's tort, such as sickness and health insurance. This would seem by some to be an unjust rule in that there is really a calculated compounding of cost and a dual recovery. The first recovery is by the payment of medical bills by the insurance companies, etc., and the second payment being the punitive damages awarded by the court.

Some argue that the phrase "punitive damages" is an unfair statement and that it is really a recompense for what has been paid for i.e., suffering, time from loss of work, etc. It is painfully evident, however, that the nature and extent of damages include emotional distress, pain, and suffering and other factors that are very difficult to quantify. The response has been to quantify them primarily on an emotional basis. In reality, one soon recognizes that the basic motivation is not only to obtain recompense for actual expenditures incurred but also as a retributive measure.

While one ordinarily thinks of punitive measures in relation to criminal law, there is no doubt that there are sufficient criteria to call this a punitive measure even in civil or equity law. An example of this is a situation where double or triple the award is given to a party because of an alleged malice or misrepresentation. Treble damages are often awarded by statute for antitrust violations. Yet another example of such a punitive measure are situations wherein the landlord of a leased property retains a security deposit. In some areas failure to properly return that security deposit results in double or triple payment back to the lessee. This borderline area, mainly the area of the landlord-tenant law, is more frequently considered a civil law action, with the addition of punitive damages. In response to this, advocacy of the "structured settlement" has met with initial success. It permits a long-term payment source based on purchase of annuities and other investment plans, thus diminishing the immediate financial impact on insurance companies, and hopefully, insurance premiums.

Some states also distribute judgments based on comparative negligence.[10] Comparative negligence is a damage apportionment system that assesses liability in proportion to fault. This approach is an alternative or replacement for the traditional doctrine of contributory negligence; it abridges but does not eliminate contributory negligence as a defense.[11]

The classical form of contributory negligence originated with Lord Ellenborough's opinion.[12] This defense was available only in situations where plaintiff's negligence was a cause of plaintiff's injuries at least in part. Traditionally, the party who was at least 51% contributorily negligent bore the full responsibility.

The Expert Witness

In medical negligence cases, the expert witness is almost indispensable. Currently, in areas of laser complications, however, we are seeing a spate of "laser experts" whose appearance for plaintiff's cases raises real questions as to expertise. The acceptance of an expert as such falls within the discretion of the presiding judge. The burden is even greater due to the relatively short time we have been using this modality and the constantly changing instrumentation and applications in the struggle against disease. Caution is urged to avoid career witnesses or organizations composed of panels of professional witnesses with minimal understanding of the physics and tissue responses related to various laser instruments and modalities and little real clinical experience.

In fact, the issue of "standard of care" still is in flux. New lasers are constantly being introduced, such as the dimer often called Encimer, exemplified by the Nd:YAG combination with krypton, and Nd:YAG combination with potassium titanite phosphate, as well as laser-activated dyes.

Standard of care usually refers to that "degree of skill, care and diligence exercised by members of the same profession, . . . in light of the present state of medical and surgical science."[13] Where technology and applications sciences advance as rapidly as with lasers, however, we must be sure that criteria of care are, in fact, established and generally accepted. Individual prejudices must not be substituted for scientific principles and controlled clinical observation. We can be helped, if only peripherally, by organizations such as the ANSI and American Society for Testing Materials, who have, on a multidisciplinary basis, addressed this issue, as well as the FDA.

REGULATORY INTERACTION

The physician is involved in regulatory considerations in three ways. First, he or she may be involved as an investigator primarily concerned with scientific research objectives, and/or funding from manufacturers for those projects. Then there is the more pervasive consideration of the impact on medical malpractice cases of FDA regulation (e.g., labeling). Similarly, those duties and responsibilities of the physician include participation on Institutional Review Boards (IRB), FDA review panels, etc.[14] We discuss these interactions and how the physician is involved.

The Investigator

As new lasers come to the fore, they must be developed under investigational device exemption parameters.[15] New instrumentation cannot move in interstate commerce unless approved by the FDA. To gain this approval, the manufacturers must submit "substantial evidence" that the device is safe and effective. This requires adequate and well-controlled investigations that ultimately involve both animal and human subjects.

The investigator first obtains approval (for human studies) from the hospital Investigational Review Board (IRB).[16] Informed consent, however burdensome, is an ethical, moral, and legal obligation. The predesigned protocol must be followed. If there is any deviation from the protocol, the entire process must be initiated anew. Adequate case histories must be documented, and the records should be retained for inspection until the entire process (study under investigational device exemption, FDA premarket approval, marketing, and statute of limitation for negligence action) is completed. The research sponsor, IRB, and FDA are all entitled to adverse effects reporting. The sponsor in turn must inform the investigator about all available preclinical studies, potential side effects, hazards, and contraindications.

The investigator *is* subject to malpractice action on the issue of "reasonableness." Keep in mind that all such suits must demonstrate that the physician-investigator did not exercise a reasonable level of skill and care (standard of care). This applies even more so to investigative procedures since, presumably, there are other approaches to therapy for the patient (including doing nothing). Food and Drug Administration approval merely signifies that the expected benefit, if any sufficiently exceeds the expected risk to render the instrument therapeutically reasonable. The *practicing* physician (clinician) is entitled to a *presumption* that a specific product can be safely and effectively used for the specific purpose studied and as approved by the FDA panel.

Investigation status is a major factor in these malpractice suits and clinicians usually argue the need for discretion in selecting therapy for their patients. Clinical investigators, however, have their discretion significantly curtailed and are specifically limited to the approved protocol.

In summary, investigational devices are limited by FDA regulations to approved investigators and for approved uses. Despite this, some individuals have been known to use investigational devices without approval or for indications outside the scope of the protocol. A prime example is the Thomas Creighton case at the University of Arizona Medical Center, Tucson (March 1985), where no attempt was made to obtain investigational device exemption approval from the FDA for the use of an artificial heart device. This recent mechanical heart transplant situation demonstrates an unnecessary apparent confrontation between the medical community and the FDA. If the developers of that particular device had initiated the IDE process, even in a less than complete manner, it is doubtful that the situation would have been as it appeared. First, section 21 C.F.R. §812.10 entitled "Waivers," allows the Agency to grant a waiver from "any requirement that FDA finds . . . is unnecessary to protect the rights, safety, or welfare of human subjects." In addition, an approved IDE can be supplemented at any time to include such changes as a new procedure involving the device or different considerations for use, etc. There *are* instances where the Agency has rapidly approved the one time or individual use of a device which had not yet received formal IDE status when it was demonstrated to be a case of dire emergency or represented the only hope for a patient. Whatever the reason, it is illegal and such practices would seem to leave the practitioner(s) and their sponsor(s) open to the full spectrum of regulatory and civil legal actions.

The initial decision as to whether or not a device constitutes a "significant risk" (defined in 21 C.F.R. §812.3 [m]) is made by the IRB, not FDA. The agency can come in after the fact and disagree with the IRB and where abuse or noncompliance occurs, the agency can require formal IDE submission even for devices that meet the conditions of the definition. What is of possible concern are the implications for practitioners and IRB panel members who are involved in the decision to use the abbreviated requirements allowed when it is decided a device meets the definition and the agency subsequently disagrees and requires formal submission of an IDE application. Such situations would put the parties involved in a weakened malpractice position.

Physician Participation on IRBs, FDA Panels, Etc.

The FDA has the responsibility, as a division of the Department of Health and Human Services, of reviewing medical devices for safety and efficacy under the Medical Device Amendments of 1976 and the Radiation Control for Health and Safety Act of 1968. To fulfill this responsibility, advisory panels have been established on which sit prominent knowledgeable physicians and other individuals. Similarly, IRBs are required for investigational uses.[17] For this work to have a salutory impact on patient care, physicians and other professionals must be willing to spend the time and effort required. Because of the implications for manufacturers, issues of conflict of interest must be avoided.[18] Therefore, FDA advisory panel members undergo a long process of selection involving extensive disclosure of assets, activities, affiliations, etc.

Disclosure of Financial Interests

> Upon completion of the clearance process you will receive an SF-50 (Notification of Personnel Action) and an HEW-410 (Supplemental Information—Expert or Consultant). It is important that you note any exclusions that may be shown on the HEW-410 in order to avoid actual, potential or appearance of conflict of interest derived from financial interests which include, but are not limited to, investments, employment, grants or contracts which you, your spouse, minor child, blood-relative residing in your household, partner, etc., may have or are negotiating.
>
> The President, May 8, 1965, issued Executive Order 11222 which requires that certain information regarding financial interest be obtained for each year of service. To facilitate updating the information each year, it is suggested you keep one copy of the FD-2637 (Confidential Statement of Employment and Financial Interests) in your files for reference purposes. If you accept new employment or obtain new financial interests prior to the annual renewal, the HHS Standards of Conduct require that you submit this information immediately. I must stress the importance of keeping your statement current. *(Personal communication.)*

It is further mandated by statute that the FDA be advised of any contracts, grants, or other monetary involvements. The obvious purpose is to assure fair and impartial expert participation. Many physicians either object to such disclosures (the confidentiality of which are protected by 21 U.S.C. §331 (j) and 18 U.S.C. §207) or are unwilling to spend the time and effort to comply. Next, there are meetings, which must be open to the concerned public under the Freedom of Information Act.[19] This means travel to Washington, D.C., for meetings. While the U.S. government does pay for travel and a small stipend for meetings, these payments are minimal. Unless the physician is willing to accept the burden as a duty to country, his or her profession and ultimately the patient or investigational subject, the public interest cannot be served. Thus, the authors recommend this "obligation" as a privilege of the profession.

The IRBs place less of a time and "red tape" burden on the physician. The review committee must recognize, accept, and conduct itself with due gravity in considering the implications of its function. Mere automatic approval of projects submitted or inaction in follow-up monitoring of projects can be disastrous for the patient or investigational subject. Political approval of projects (you approve my proposals today so that I will approve yours tomorrow) cannot be accepted as a matter of integrity, professionalism, and the public welfare. In addition, this risks legal action in event of injury to the subject-patient. We must keep in mind that these committee members, the institution, and the investigational team are all liable for injuries produced. These committees are not usually legally protected by peer review statutes. (Note: peer review statutes usually protect *post hoc* review committees from legal liability to reviewed individuals. The public interest aspect is to provide a mechanism for quality control of patient care and investigational practices.)

In summary, we do need top-notch physicians, cognizant of their moral, ethical, and legal obligations for investigational premarket approval and medical device peer review committees.

PRODUCT LIABILITY

Product liability is another area of tort law to be considered briefly. It is usually described as the responsibility of the manufacturer to those individuals who can reasonably be expected to use the products so manufactured. It encompasses not only those who the manufacturer intended to purchase the instrumentation, but also those who, while unintended, might ultimately come into possession of or be injured by, the modality.[20] The physician *is* a peripheral participant.

The manufacturer may be liable for mistakes in design, manufacture, testing, failure to warn, or in contract for breach of statutory or common law warranties (of merchantability or fitness for purpose intended) or in strict liability for marketing a defective product.[21] The courts will impose liability on a doctor or hospital where there is proof of misuse of the device *or continued use* of the device in the face of known or reasonably discoverable defects[22] or negligent selection of the particular device for the task at hand.[23] Additionally, the courts will impose a duty to inspect devices before use. The application of these principles should be self evident in the case of laser instrumentation.

The question of whether physicians and hospitals should be held liable under the theory of *strict liability* (no-fault) in tort has been addressed by some commentators.[24] The rationale for this has been the *deep pocket theory*. The party who is injured as a result of a defective product usually is unable to bear the financial consequences. The source of financial retribution (physicians and hospitals with financial resources, including impersonal insurance coverage) therefore becomes the target. Fortunately, most state courts[25] have rejected this extension so far.

A concept closely related to that of "strict liability" is "res ipsa loquitur." Under this evidentiary doctrine a presumption of negligence on the part of a defendant may be raised where it can be shown that the instrument that caused the harm was under the control and management of the defendant, and that the accident would not have occurred in the ordinary course of affairs if the defendant had used proper care. In some cases courts have applied this doctrine against the physician and hospital even where it was *possible* that the manufacturer was the culpable party.[26] A different approach was taken by the Supreme Court of New Jersey,[27] stating that (338 A. 2d @ 7) "the *burden of proof* (emphasis added by author) in fact does shift to defendants. All those in custody of that patient or who owed him a duty, . . . should be called forward and should be made to prove their freedom from liability."

In fact, a physician or hospital may be liable for the following: (a) negligent misuse of a device; (b) negligent selection of a device; (c) failure to inspect or test the device, and (d) using the device with knowledge of its being defective.

These four theories of failure of duty are clearly applicable to practitioners of the laser art, with particular emphasis on items (c) and (d). A practical example is the situation wherein the surgeon assumes the laser to be in focus without so testing it *before each case* or at least each day. Liability for failure to make reasonable testing or inspection for latent defects may be the prime basis for legal action.[28] Similarly, though perhaps worthy of greater condemnation, is the circumstance where there is foreknowledge of a dissimilarity between the focusing He-Ne indicator beam and the actual CO_2 burn site. The use of this latter instrument thus is rampant with risk to the patient and liability for the physician, hospital, and their agents. An analogous situation, yet to be tested, is proceeding with administration of an anesthetic by the anesthesiologist with full knowledge that the surgeon has not yet tested the laser for focus and function (including sufficient gas). In the event the machine malfunctions, and an alternate approach is not immediately available (e.g., in the case of stenosis of the trachea), and the patient is shown to have thereby been injured by either the malfunction or an "unnecessary" anesthetic, legal risk may accrue to all parties concerned.

Another option available to the plaintiff is the legal concept of joinder.

Here, the physician is charged with negligence in use of an instrument, but this time the physician is joined by another alleged culprit—the manufacturer of the laser. This joinder of the laser manufacturer is an example of how, until recently, the applicability of products liability concepts to medical malpractice has been largely ignored.[29]

The most interesting defense for the manufacturer is product misuse. If the products-liability defendant establishes misuse by the physician, a case of malpractice will also be convincingly established. If the plaintiff does not prevail on his or her products-liability concepts theory due to the product misuse defense, his or her negligence theory against a defendant physician has been enhanced. Thus the plaintiff patient is in a "can't lose" situation and the surgeon "can't win." A prototype of this scenario was *Ethicon, Inc. vs. Parten,*[30] where the product misuse defense was raised. The court granted a directed verdict for the physician and the hospital in all negligence actions and cross-actions for misuse against the physician and the hospital by the manufacturer seeking contribution and indemnity. The court indicated that the burden of proof required to establish a right to contribution or indemnity would be the same as in a case for medical malpractice.[31] Thus, while the physician, who stands in a position of special trust and responsibility, may endanger the welfare of his or her patient because of misuse of a medical instrument, he or she may also place the manufacturer in a position of liability. In so doing, he or she may expect the manufacturer (in self-interest) to proceed and act against him or her legally.

There is a trend developing in this era of Diagnostic Related Groupings (DRGs) and TEFRA[32] that potentially increases risk management problems for hospitals and some physician managers. This relates to service contracts provided by manufacturers. The manufacturers' or distributors' service contracts are quite expensive. Therefore, some maintenance departments and individuals do in-house maintenance and servicing equipment. What now appears as a less expensive alternative to service contracts may turn out to be a costly choice (a pyrrhic victory). The automobile industry is the classic example of this legal defense argumentation by manufacturers' counsel. In the medical instrument context, the issue would be whether the hospital assigned as their agent a maintenance or repair person who was properly trained and skilled to handle the specific device (i.e., laser). Of course, "where an act of negligence is a substantial factor in bringing about an injury, it does not cease to be a legal and proximate cause thereof because of the intervention of a subsequent act of negligence of another which contributed to the injury, if the prior act of negligence is still operating, and the injury inflicted is not different in kind from that which would have resulted from the prior act."[33] Manufacturers of equipment tend to shift the blame on the theory that the appropriate care in utilizing, maintaining, and repair was not taken.[34] The plaintiff need only show that defendant hospital had care, control, or custody of the laser at the time the negligent risk was created by utilizing the services of its inadequately trained maintenance personnel.[35] The key to this approach is that while "intervening negligence" may not insulate the manufacturer entirely, it expands the defendant pool to include the hospital, physicians, or other personnel who were involved in assigning the inadequately trained maintenance person and with the additional theory of breach of "implied warranty to fitness for use intended."[36]

The complexity of the above argumentation reflects the many interrelationships in medical practice between patient, manufacturer, and practitioner of medicine.

We have presented herein some of the highlights of the manifold relationships in the medical device field. Physicians, hospitals, and manufacturers interact in bringing their respective products to the service of the patient. The introduction of lasers in patient care is a prime example of these relationships—and responsibilities.

REFERENCES AND CITATIONS

1. Federal Food, Drug and Cosmetic Act of 1938; Medical Device Amendments of 1976; H.R. Rep. No. 94-853, 94th Cong., 2d Sess. (1976) as amended; 21 CFR; Laws Enforced by the U.S. Food and Drug Administration (1981); Radiation Control for Health and Safety Act, 1968; 42 U.S.C.; 18 U.S.C. and FOIA 5 U.S.C., as well as pertinent Office of Management and Budget and U.S. Customs Provisions and Occupational Safety and Health Act of 1970, P.L. 91-596 (1970), 29 U.S.C.A. SS 651 *et seq.*
2. *Lipscomb v. Memorial Hospital,* 733 F. 2d 232, 336 (4th Cir. 1984); *Canterbury v. Spence,* U.S. Ct. App. for the D.C. Cir., 1972, 150 U.S. App. D.C. 263, 464 F. 2d 772 (1972); certiorari denied, 409 U.S. 1064, 93 S. Ct. 560, 34 L.Ed. 2d 518.
3. *Hartke v. McKelway,* 707 F. 2d 1544, 1549–50 (D.C. Cir.) *cert. denied,* 104 S. Ct. 425 (1983).
4. *Schloendorf v. Society of N.Y. Hospital,* 211 N.Y. 125, 105 N.E. 92 (1914).
5. *Martha Logan v. Greenwich Hospital Association et al.,* Conn. Sup. Ct., No. 10969, Sept. 6, 1983.
6. *Bowen v. Iȯwa Nat. Mut. Ins. Co.,* 270 N.C. 486, 155 S.E. 2d 238, 242 (1967).
7. Norton M.L.: When Does an Experimental/Innovative Procedure Become an Accepted Procedure? *The Pharos of Alpha Omega Alpha* 38:4, 161–165, Oct. 1973.
8. Ladimer I.: Ethical and legal aspects of medical research in human beings. *J. Pub. Law* 3:467, 1954; Ladimer I.: Human experimentation: Medicolegal aspects. *N. Engl. J. Med.* 256:18, 1957.
9. *Kirtland & Packard v. Superior Court for County of Los Angeles,* 59 Cal. App. 3d 140, 131 Cal. Rptr. 418, 421; Helfend v. Southern Cal. Rapid Transit Disc., 84 Cal. Rptr. 73, 2 Cal. 3d 1, 465 P. 2d 61, 73 (1970).

10. *Placek v. City of Sterling Heights,* 405 Mich. 638, 275 N.W. 2d 511, 527–528 (1979).
11. *West v. Caterpillar Tractor Co.,* 336 So. 2d 80, 90 (Fla. 1976); see also *Butand v. Suburban Marine and Sporting Goods, Inc.,* 555 P. 2d 42 (Alaska 1976).
12. *Butterfield v. Forrester,* 103 Eng. Rep. 926 (1809).
13. *Gillette v. Tucker,* 67 Ohio St. 106, 65 N.E. 865, (1902); see also *Bruni v Tatsumi,* 46 Ohio St. 2d 127, 129, 346 N.E. 2d 673, 676 (1976).
14. Federal Advisory Committee Act; Publ. No. 92-463, 86 Stat. 770 (1972); Kahan J.S., Medical Lasers and the Law, Medical Device and Diagnostic Injury, 6:11, 83–85, 118–119 (Nov. 1984); Kahan J.S., Gibbs J.N., The Impact on Medical Malpractice Cases of Food and Drug Administration Regulation, submitted for publication (1985); Kahan J.S., Laser and Electronic Medical Devices—An Overview of Food and Drug Administration Regulation, 38 Food and Drug Cosmetic L.J. 220 (1983).
15. 21 CFR 812.140–812.150.
16. Schwartz, E.: Institutional Review of Medical Research, 4 J. Legal Med. 143 (1983).
17. 21 C.F.R. Part 56, 1984.
18. Standards of Conduct, 45 CFR Part 73; Fed. Reg. 46:15, 7368–7385.
19. Freedom Of Information Act, 5 U.S.C. S 552; see also Fed. Advisory Committee 5 U.S.C. S 901 *et seq.*
20. Restatement (Second) of Torts, Sect. 402A, subsect 2a and b; *Bowles v. Zimmer Mfg. Co.,* 277 F2d 868 (7th Cir. 1960) applying Michigan law; *Ribando v. Amer. Cyanamid Co.,* 37 Misc. 2d 603, 235 N.Y.S. 2d 110 (Sup. Ct. 1962).
21. Rubin, Manufacturer and Professional Users Liability for Defective Medical Equipment, 8 Akron L. Rev. 1, 99, 110 (1974).
22. *Shepard v. McGinnis,* 257 Iowa 35, 131 N.W. 2d 475 (1964).
23. *Phillips v. Powell,* 290 P. 441 (Cal. 1930).
24. Russell, "Product and the Professional: Strict Liability in the Sales-Service Hybrid Transaction", 24 Hastings L.J. 111 (1972); *see also* "The Medical Profession and Strict Liability for Defective Products—A Limited Extension", 17 Hastings L.J. 350 (1965).
25. *Silverhart v. Mount Zion Hospital,* 20 Cal. App. 3d 1022, 98 Cal. Rptr. 187 (1971); *Magrine v. Krasnica* 94 N.J. Super. 228, 227 A. 2d 539 (1967), aff'd. sub nom., *Magrine v. Spector,* 100 N.J. Super. 223, 241 A 2d 637 (App. Div. 1968), aff'd. 53 N.J. 259, 250 A. 2d 129 (1969).
26. *Dierman v. Providence Hospital,* 31 Cal. 2d 290, 188 P2d 12 (1947).
27. *Anderson v. Somberg,* 67 N.J. 291, 338 A 2d 1, *cert. denied,* 423 U.S. 929 (1975).
28. *Tenant v. Barton,* 164 Wash. 279, 2P. 2d 735 (1931); Stafford v. St. Clair's Hospital 19 Misc. 2d 710, 187 N.Y.S. 2d 351 (Sup. Ct. 1959).
29. Frumer and Friedman, Products Liability S 34A (1978).
30. *Ethicon, Inc. v. Parten,* 520 S.W. 2d 527 (Tex. Civ. App.—Houston [14th Dist.] 1975).
31. *Bowles v. Bourden,* 219 S.W. 2d 779 (Tex. 1949).
32. Tax Equity and Fiscal Responsibility Act of 1982; P.L. 97–248.
33. 2 Restatement, Torts, SS 440–442, 447.

34. 18 Def. L.J. 196 (1969) summarizing defendant's arguments in *O'Brien v. Yoder Co.* (W.D. Wis. 1968).
35. *Hanberry v. Hearst Corp.,* 81 Cal. Rptr. 519, Ct. of App. Fourth Dist., 1 Cal. App. 3d 149 (1969).
36. *Connoly v. Hagi,* 24 Conn. Sup. Ct. 198, 188 A 2d 884 (1963).

13 The Future of Laser Surgery of the Head and Neck

Marvin P. Fried, M.D.

The introduction of the operating microscope to clinical laryngology changed the surgeon's perspective on disease. Not only was the obvious advantage of magnification achieved, but also the degree of precision was greatly improved. Biopsy could be more appropriate, and small lesions could be resected without sacrificing normal adjacent structures, thereby minimizing scar and functional alterations. As magnification increased, instrumentation became smaller, but it was not until the advent of the surgical laser that a major new stride in laryngology was taken. Although basically a light scalpel, the properties of the laser added a new dimension to the surgery of the aerodigestive tract. Foremost of these advantages was cutting precision commensurate with improved visualization. Improved "seeing" and improved "doing" were coupled. These benefits have been discussed in chapter 1 by Dr. Strome. Once established, improvements in laser instrument design and application were accomplished by many interested groups including physicians, physicists, bioelectric engineers, and manufacturers. This broad approach to laser technology and surgery has assured rapid growth and change. It is difficult to view the future with all of this current activity, but certain directions have already been established.

THE FUTURE IN LASER INSTRUMENTATION

One obvious advance that has become apparent is the attempt to reduce the size of the laser housing system. This affords increased mobility within the operating suite as well as at the microscope level. Limits exist due to the size of the laser tube and most modifications have taken place with the

CO_2 units. Housing designs have placed the laser at or in the microscope stand as well as at the console. In either case, articulating devices remain clumsy and cumbersome, limiting motion of the microscope. Miniaturization of the umbilical cables will improve this flexibility.

With smaller units, the laser can be brought closer to the operative field. The capability to develop these devises depends greatly on how the laser beam is transported. As noted before, this currently limits flexibility from source to the surgeon's hand. This also limits delivery to the tissue. A practical fiberoptic cable that can transmit a CO_2 laser seems to be close to perfection and would allow this next phase of development to occur. Current Nd:YAG lasers use fiberoptic cables, but access to tissue is still by rigid endoscopes. Moreover, the depth of penetration by the YAG laser is variable, limiting its utility. A CO_2 fiberoptic delivery system will allow access to not only the distal tracheobronchial tree, but also many regions in the head and neck. The point of emission of the laser beam could also be placed at the end of instruments, providing a shorter working distance and less of a margin for error. The amalgamation of the tasks of visualization, cutting or ablation, suction and coagulation into a single instrument would then be practical.

The trend, now beginning, to decreased spot size will probably continue. This will increase the power density at a single point, thus enabling CO_2 laser units to be built with diminished power (watt) output. If larger resections are needed, or application of the same laser unit to gynecology and neurosurgery, the range of varying spot size and power can be advantageous. Additional applications of reduced spot size are mentioned below. Increased power used over a broad field may enable rapid tumor ablation, but runs the risk of scatter of tumor cells. This area in particular will require thorough laboratory investigation prior to clinical application.

With laser miniaturization will come the likely integration of various laser source units into one system. The use of multiple wavelength sources will allow for varied penetration, selective effect in various tissues within an organ as well as selection of incisions, coagulation, fusion, or ablation. Additional sources will be perfected with capabilities beyond those thought of today as well as methods to increase laser specificity. One method that has already progressed to clinical application is laser photoradiation therapy employing the photosensitizing agent, hematoporphyrin derivative (HPD) or dihematoporphyrin ether (DHE). Dougherty[1] had demonstrated that this agent could be selectively retained by tumor cells. When these cells are illuminated with red light (630 nm), the HPD absorbs the light-producing photodynamic action that results in tumor destruction. Singlet oxygen is thought to be the agent that ultimately causes cell death, and is generated as a result of light interaction with a component of HPD (probably DHE).

Singlet oxygen impairs cell membrane function and integrity by oxidation. Normal tissues are not damaged. The light is usually derived from an argon laser–driven dye laser. This "fine tuning" of laser action has found application in tumors of the tracheobronchial tree, prostate, and skin, as well as the head and neck. The concepts of selective identification and destruction of tissue components could be enhanced in the future with the nuclear magnetic resonance scanners that may aid in diagnosis by cell type and composition. The appropriate photosensitizing agent can then be given and the corresponding wavelength laser applied. Normal tissue would be spared and massive ablation and subsequent reconstruction would be avoided.

THE FUTURE IN LASER APPLICATION

The CO_2 laser still finds its greatest head and neck application in the airway. With fiberoptic cables distal sites can be reached. Illumination will be brighter, as will the aiming beam to increase precision, even before the ablating laser is turned on. Access to the sinonasal tract will be improved, perhaps with intrasinus surgery, avoiding radical sinusotomy and wall destruction. Choanal atresia may be corrected by the transnasal approach. Similarly, the sphenoid sinus and pituitary can be approached under direct endoscopic visualization and radiographic monitoring.

The laser, no matter what the energy source, is ideally suited for otologic surgery. Integration within the microscope would provide for incision, as well as welding the tympanic membrane and middle ear structures. Cholesteatoma can be removed leaving adjacent normal tissue undisturbed. Thin (less than 1 mm) fiberoptic cables can carry surgery into the labyrinth, allowing selective destruction of specific semicircular canals, saccule, or utricle. Neurinomas can be "peeled" from the trunks of the facial and acoustic nerves.

Intravascular laser application may find a role in restoring patency to vessels not only serving the heart, but in other sites as well. Increased precision in the vertebral-basilar system could diminish the occurrence of vertigo due to this common cause. Even small vessels, such as those supplying the cochlea may be reached, thus reversing what now seems to be one reason for sudden hearing loss.

Vascular surgery can be aided in other ways using the laser. Microspot lasers (using low power) will be able to fuse both arteries and veins, performing anastomoses that now require sutures. Less trauma would be transmitted to the endothelium, increasing the patency rate, as well as diminishing the time it takes to perform the anastomosis. Nerves as well can be joined, sealing the epineurium and thereby decreasing the likelihood for neuroma formation by preventing the sprouting of axons outside of the anastomosis.

Pigmented lesions of the skin, including melanoma, will continue to be treated with the laser, with different colors "tuned" to specific wavelengths.

Currently, as well as for the foreseeable future, advances in laser technology may far precede the clinical applications. Defining the appropriate role of the laser when compared with standard techniques will require imagination and continued monitoring of efficacy and safety.

THE FUTURE IN LASER SAFETY

The application of the laser to new tasks requires careful evaluation of potential hazards. Laboratory experimentation must assess these risks as well as the means to avoid them. As more laser units are developed, marketed, and purchased, greater numbers of surgeons will use them. These individuals will require training and possible certification. Training must include not only lectures, but also "hands-on" experience either through residency programs or surgical courses. Whether certification will be on an individual course or hospital basis or even by a national organization will need to be decided.

Standards for manufacturing of instruments are being developed with assistance by the American National Standards Institute (ANSI). This will assure some uniformity in design and classification of instruments.

Guidelines for safe laser usage in various specialties will also be suggested, but supervision of these recommendations will be difficult and will probably need to be adopted in an individual hospital or surgical center basis. This will also lead to the question of the appropriate site for laser surgery. Up to this time, most laser surgery is performed in a hospital setting. With the current pressures to perform more operations on an ambulatory basis, laser surgery will follow as well. Risks, particularly within the first few hours following surgery, will have to be carefully defined so that no untoward events ensue.

Modification in equipment will surely involve development of nonflammable endotracheal tubes as well as heat resistant fiberoptic cables. Gas mixtures, such as helium-oxygen,[2] will allow increased heat absorption and less fires. With smaller laser spot size, more normal tissue will be spared. This would also be the benefit with selective laser absorption. Improved depth control will produce the same effect.

The potentials for the future are numerous and with closer association of all groups involved in laser design, research, manufacture, and application, the development as well as safety of the laser will progress concomitantly.

REFERENCES

1. Dougherty T.J., Grindley G.B., Fiel R., et al.: Photoradiation therapy: II. Care of animal tumors with hematoporphyrin and light. *J. Natl. Cancer Instit.* 55:115–121, 1975.
2. Cassissi N.J., Pashayan A.G., Gravenstein J.S.: Helium-oxygen mixture (Gator gas) prevents laser fires. Presented at the annual meeting of the American Academy of Otolaryngology–Head and Neck Surgery, Las Vegas, 1984.

Appendix A Laser Safety Regulations: University of Michigan

CHARGE

A process to credential physicians at University of Michigan Hospitals.

RECOMMENDATION

A. Delineation of Clinical Privileges by each service will be initiated by the individual desiring such privileges who will certify to the respective Chairman or Chief of the department, section and/or division that he/she fulfills the recommended guidelines. The Chairman or Chief or designee, reviews the application and provides prior authorization and approval of credentials, certifying same to the Credentials Committee. The Credentials Committee will then review the Chairman's/Chief's certification and notify appropriate offices (including the certification and notify appropriate offices (including the LSO). The Committee will keep a file of approved individuals with credentials in laser application.

B. Recommended guidelines for Laser Credential approval:
   1. Demonstrated understanding of laser physics, power density, and laser tissue interaction.
   2. Experience in animal laboratory as preparation for patient experience.
   3. Demonstrated formal course "hands-on" training.

      and/or

   4. Experience and approval in patient application under direct and immediate supervision of trained operator of the laser.

5. The requisite experience must be related to the specific class of instrument to be used. (NOTE: It is dangerous to assume that all instruments are alike or that all media [CO_2, Nd:YAG, argon, ruby, erbium, etc.] are the same in effect.)

C. Recommended: (a) general training to be provided by each department, section and/or division to employees working with or around lasers stressing safety and operational hazards; (b) development of institutional laser safety training program to include:
1. Fundamentals of laser operation (physical principles, construction, etc.).
2. Bioeffects of laser radiation.
3. Relations of specular and diffuse reflections.
4. Nonradiation hazards (electrical, chemical, reaction by-products, etc.).
5. Control methods.
6. Overall management and responsibilities.
7. Medical surveillance practices.
8. Ancillary problems in laser usage (airway management, etc.).

CHARGE

To develop institutional laser safety standards for both outpatient and inpatient laser use at University of Michigan Hospitals.

RECOMMENDATION

A. All personnel shall wear safety eye glasses (appropriate to the laser) with *side guards*.

B. When performing head and neck surgery, laser application, the patient's eyes and contiguous tissue or flammable substrate shall be covered with wet eye pads and *canvas* tape that must be kept wet throughout the procedures, or other appropriate protective measures. Special attention shall be paid to keep the other areas around the operating table (floor, foot switch, etc.) dry, including sites of potential skin contact. The operator of the laser system must take special precautions when operating, adjusting, or modifying power input or laser cabinet (*see also* item N below) to avoid risk of electroshock, potential electrocution, or electrical burns.

C. The laser is not to be used in the presence of flammables or combustibles (i.e., anesthetics, prep solutions, drying agents, ointments, methyl methacrylate, or other plastics). Wet cloth towels should be used to drape the immediate area instead of plastic or paper drapes.

D. A master control key is necessary for operation of the laser. Only personnel qualified to use and operate the laser shall have access to this key. The key should be removed when the laser is not in operation.

E. The supervising operating laser surgeon must remain in the room at *all* times when the laser is in use.

F. Signs shall be posted on *all* doors entering the laser suite stating that laser use is in progress. Only personnel directly involved in care of the patient will be permitted in the room, except by special permission of the operator. Current policy requires approval of the Administration Director, or designee, as well.

G. The laser machine will remain OFF when not in use, including in the operating room after testing. The "standby mode" should be permitted only for very brief periods when adjusting the power meter and/or using other short-term instrumentation.

H. Only the operating surgeon shall operate the laser activating switch or power control.

I. Where available, instrumentation should be provided that will defract, scatter, or defocus the beam rather than reflect or focus it elsewhere.

J. During surgery in the aerodigestive tract (oral, nasopharyngeal, laryngotracheal, or endobronchial), the endotracheal tube, where used, must be protected. Anesthesia personnel must use nonflammable endotracheal tubes (e.g., Hirschman or Norton) or specially wrapped red rubber or *100%* silicone (e.g., Milhaud Nitrogen protected) tubes. Other plastics, portex, anode (wired, armored) tubes (even if wrapped) must never be used. The inflated cuff and length of tubes must be protected.

K. Intracavitary laser applications outside the operating suite will require *prior* scheduling availability of the operating room (or comparable ADSU facility) to manage complications.

L. When the indicator (visible) laser beam is not in absolute conformity with surgical laser beam (e.g., CO_2 burn site), the instrument is NOT to be used and shall be repaired before use on the patient.

M. For a laser that requires water cooling, a suitable source and drain shall be available. The characteristics of the source and drain shall meet the requirements of the laser as specified by the manufacturer. Parameters normally required are minimum flow rate that must be maintained, maximum input temperature allowed for sufficient cooling, and the reliability of the water source including any alarms that may be necessary if it is interrupted.

N. The electrical supply for the laser must meet the requirements stated by the manufacturer. The frequency, voltage, and power requirements are expected to be within the electrical service normally provided; hence, in most cases, no special wiring will be required. In the event the laser requires a unique power source, Hospital Plant Engineering can be issued a work order to install it to the manufacturer's specifications. All lasers should be provided with a ground for the case of the instrument. This ground is normally part of the electrical supply.

O. Ventilatory requirements in the room fall into two categories:
   1. Ventilation necessary to keep the laser cool, and to remove any gases or vapors that may be inherent in laser operation.
   2. Ventilation necessary to remove gases or vapors that are produced by the effect of the laser beam on tissues involved in the medical procedure.

   It is expected that the normal room ventilation and/or the suction equipment usually provided in the procedure room will be adequate in most instances. The manufacturer's recommendation should be made available for no. 1 above. Medical procedures should determine the ventilation or suction requirements for no. 2 above. Such ventilation may not be part of the laser instruction books.

P. Anesthesia guidelines for laser procedures will be established according to ANSI standards Z 136.3.

CHARGE

A monitoring system at the University of Michigan Hospitals to assure the standards are being met.

RECOMMENDATION

A. Designation of a *Laser Safety Officer* (LSO) for the Institution from among such personnel as are regularly within the institution and immediately available during laser procedures.

   Duties

   1. The LSO will have authority to supervise the control of laser

hazards. The LSO will provide consultative services on laser hazard evaluation and controls, and on personnel training programs.

2. The LSO will have the authority to approve, suspend, restrict, or terminate the operation of a laser or laser system if the LSO deems that laser hazard controls are inadequate.
3. The LSO will ensure that necessary records required are maintained, and will maintain records of individuals authorized to work with lasers in the medical context, and a file of known or suspected accidents.
4. When a known or suspected laser-related accident is brought to the attention of the LSO, this will be brought to the attention of the Chairman or Chief of the respective department, seciton, and/or division, and, if indicated, the Risk Management Section and/or other appropriate institutional offices.

B. Designation, by Chairman or Chief of respective department, section, and/or division utilizing the laser, of a Deputy Laser Safety Officer for that department, section, and/or division who will perform the functions of the LSO for that unit, and report to the Institutional LSO, as well as the respective Chairman or Chief, in which case the LSO or Chairman or Chief will take appropriate action.

C. Designation of a continuing Laser Safety Committee to serve in an advisory capacity to the LSO, who shall be a member of that committee. The committee will establish and maintain adequate policies and regulations and recommend the appropriate laser safety training programs, and maintain an awareness and incorporate new or revised laser safety standards as appropriate.

D. Maintenance, repair, and testing policies will fall in the purview of the designated Deputy LSO of the Department of Plant Engineering. No laser system will be released for use until approved by the Department of Plant Engineering.

Appendix B | Glossary of Legal Terminology

Martin L. Norton, M.D., J.D.

Edward V. Norton, J.D.

The definitional appendix noted herein has been derived primarily, though not solely, from *Black's Law Dictionary,* ed. 5, St. Paul, Minn., West Publishing Co., 1979.

Actionable Tort

To constitute an "actionable tort" there must be a legal duty imposed by statute or otherwise owing by the defendant to the one injured and in the absence of such duty damage caused is "injury without wrong" or "damnum absque injuria."

Coleman v. California Yearly Meeting of Friends Church, 27 Cal. App. 2d 579, 81 P. 2d 469, 470. (1938)

Agency

Agency is the fiduciary relation which results from the manifestation of consent by one person to another that the other shall act on his behalf and subject to his control, and consent by the other so to act.

Restatement (Second) of Agency §1.

Agent

A person authorized by another to act for him, who is entrusted with another's business.

Humphries v. Going, 59 F.R.D. 583, 587 (D.C.N.C. 1972).

Apparent or Ostensible Agent

One whom the principal, either intentionally or by want of ordinary care, induces third persons to believe to be his agent, though he has not either expressly or by implication conferred authority on him. A person who, whether or not authorized, reasonably appears to the third person because of manifestations of another, to be authorized to act as an agent for such other person.

Restatement (Second) of Agency §8.

Burden of Proof

In the law of evidence, the necessity or duty of affirmatively proving a fact or fact-in-dispute on an issue raised between the parties in a cause of legal action. The obligation of a party to establish by evidence a requisite degree of belief concerning a fact in mind of the trier effect or the court.

Cause of Action

The fact or facts which give a person a right to judicial relief. The fact or a state of facts to which the law is sought to be enforced against a person or thing applies. Facts which give rise to one or more relations of right/duty between two or more persons.

Thompson v. Zurich Insurance Co., (D. Minn. 1970), 309 F. Supp. 1178, 1181.

Comparative Negligence

Negligence measured in terms of percentage with damages allowed diminished in proportion to amount of negligence.

Consent

Consent is an act of reason accompanied with deliberation, weighing in the balance the good or evil on each side. It means voluntary agreement by a person in the possession and exercise of sufficient mental capacity to make an intelligent choice to do something proposed by another. Consent is implied in every agreement. It is an act unclouded by unflawed duress or sometimes even mistake.

Contributory Negligence

The act or omission amounting to want of ordinary care on part of complaining party, which, concurring with defendant's negligence is proximate cause of injury.

Honaker v. Crutchfield, 247 Ky 495, 57 S.W. 2d 502 (Ct. App. 1933).

Culpable

Involving the breach of a legal duty or the commission of a fault.

Duty

In negligence cases the term may be defined as an obligation to which law will give recognition and effect to conform to a particular standard of conduct towards another.

Rasmussen v. Prudential Insurance Co., 277 Minn. 266, 152 N.W. 2d 359, 362 (1967).

The word "duty" is used throughout Restatement of Torts to denote the fact that the actor is required to conduct himself in a particular manner at the risk that if he does not do so he becomes subject to liability to another to whom the duty is owed for any injury sustained by such other of which the actor's conduct is a legal cause.

Restatement (Second) of Torts §4.

Equity

The spirit and habit of fairness, justice and right dealing which would regulate the relationships of men with men.

Giles v. Dept. of Human Resources Development, 11 Cal. 3d 313, 113 Cal. Rptr. 374, 380, 521 P. 2d 110 (1974).

Expert Testimony

Opinion evidence of some person who possesses special skill or knowledge in some science profession or business which is not common to the average man and which is possessed by the expert by reason of his special study or experience.

Board of Educ. of Claymont Special School Dist. v. 13 Acres of land in Brandywine Hundred, 11 Terry 387, 131 A. 2d 180, 184 (Del. Super. Ct. 1950).

Fiduciary Relation

A fiduciary relation arises whenever confidence is reposed on one side and domination and influence result on the other. The relation can be legal, social, domestic or merely personal.

Matter of Estate of Hellman, 37 Ill. App. 3d 390, 345 N.E. 2d 536, 540 (1976).

Such relationship exists when there is a reposing of faith, confidence and trust and the placing of reliance by one upon the judgment and advise of the other.

Williams v. Griffin, 35 Mich. App. 179, 192 N.W. 2d 283, 285 (1971).

Out of such a relation, the law raises the rule that neither party may exert influence or pressure upon the other, take selfish advantage of his trust or deal with the subject matter of the trust in such a way as to benefit himself or prejudice the other except in the exercise of the utmost good faith and with the full knowledge and consent of the other.

Implied Consent

That consent manifested by signs, actions or facts, or by inaction or silence which raise a presumption that the consent has been given.

Implied Contract

Implied contracts are those wherein the obligations are imposed upon a person, either express or implied, because the circumstances between the parties are such as to render it just, that the one should have a right, and the other a corresponding liability similar to those which would arise from a contract between them. There can be no true contract without a mutual and concurrent intention of the parties, however. Such obligations are more properly described as "quasi contracts."

Joinder of Parties

The act of uniting as parties to an action all persons who have claimed the same rights or against whom rights are claimed as either co-plaintiffs or co-defendants.

Fed. R. Civil P. 19 and 20.

Joint and Several Contracts

Contracts in which the parties bind themselves individually and as a unit jointly.

Joint and Several Liability

A liability is said to be joint and several when the plaintiff may sue one or more of the parties to such liability separately, or all of them together at his option.

Joint Tortfeasors

This term refers to two or more persons jointly or severally liable in tort for the same injury to person or property. This includes those who act together in committing a wrong or whose acts, if independent of each other, unite in causing a single injury.

American Tobacco Co. v. Transport Corp., 277 F. Supp. 457, 461 (E.D.Va. 1957); *Bowen v. Iowa National Mutual Insurance Co.,* 270 N.C. 486, 155 S.E. 2d 238, 242 (1967).

Liable

Bound or obliged in law or equity; responsible, chargeable, answerable, compellable to make satisfaction, compensation or restitution.

Homan v. Employers Reinsurance Corp., 345 Mo. 650, 136 S.W. 2d 289, 298 (1939).

Malpractice

Any professional misconduct, unreasonable lack of skill or fidelity in professional or fiduciary duties, evil malpractice or illegal or immoral conduct.

Matthews v. Walker, 34 Ohio App. 2d 128, 296 N.E. 2d 569, 577, 63 O.O. 2d 208 (1973). See Also *Kosberg v. Wash. Hosp. Center Inc.,* 129 U.S. App. D.C. 322, 394 F. 2d 947, 949 (1968).

Negligence

Negligence is the failure to use such care as a reasonably prudent and careful person would use under similar circumstances. It is the doing of some act which a person of ordinary prudence would not have done under similar circumstances or failure to do what a person of ordinary prudence would have done under similar circumstances.

Amoco Chemical Corp. v. Hill, 318 A. 2d 614, 617 (Del. Super. Ct. 1974).

Ordinary Care

That degree of care which ordinarily prudent and competent persons engaged in the same line of business or endeavor should exercise under similar circumstances, and in law means same as "due care" and "reasonable care."

Warner v. Kiowa County Hospital Authority, Okl. App., 551 P. 2d 1179, 1188 (Okla. App. Ct. 1976).

That care which reasonably prudent persons exercise in the management of their own affairs in order to avoid injury to themselves or their property or the persons or property of others.

Post Facto

From the Latin, after the fact.

Proximate Cause

That which in a natural and continuous sequence unbroken by any efficient intervening cause produces injury and without which the result would not have occurred. That which stands next in causation to the effect, not necessarily in time or space but in causal relation. The proximate cause of any injury is the primary or moving cause, or that which in a natural and continuous sequence, unbroken by any efficient intervening cause produces the injury and without which the accident could not have happened if the injury be one which might be reasonably anticipated or foreseen as natural consequence of the wrongful act. It has also been defined as the dominant moving or producing cause, the efficient cause; the one that necessarily sets the other causes in operation.

Herron v. Smith Bros., 116 Cal. App. 518, 2 P. 2d 1012, 1013 (1931).

Reliance

This term is used in the rule imposing liability on one who volunteers to undertake action for the protection of another person or things for failure to exercise reasonable care if harm is suffered because of the other's reliance upon the undertaking. The term connotes dependence, it implies a voluntary choice of conduct by the person harmed and infers that the person exercising it can decide between available alternatives.

Barnum v. Rural Fire Protection Co., 24 Ariz. App. 233, 537 P. 2d 618, 622 (1975). See also, *Gordon v. Burr,* D.C. N.Y., 366 F. Supp. 156, 165 (S.D.N.Y. 1973).

Res Ipsa Loquitur

The rule of evidence whereby negligence of an alleged wrongdoer may be inferred from the mere fact that the accident happened provided that the character of accident and the circumstances attending it lead reasonably to the belief that in the absence of negligence it would not have occurred and that the thing which caused injury is shown to have been under the management and control of the alleged wrongdoer.

Hillen v. Hooker Construction Co., Tex. Civ. App. 484 S.W. 2d 113, 115 (1972).

Under the doctrine of "res ipsa loquitur" the happening of an injury permits an inference of negligence where the plaintiff produces substantial evidence that the injury was caused by an agency or instrumentality under the exclusive control and management of the defendant and that the occurrence was such that in the ordinary course of things would not happen if reasonable care had been used.

Standard of Care

In medical, legal, etc., malpractice cases, a standard of care is applied to measure the competence of the professional. The traditional standard for doctors is that he exercise the average degree of skill, care, and diligence, exercised by members of the same profession practicing in the same or a similar locality in light of the present state of medical and surgical science.

Gillette v. Tucker, 67 Ohio St. 106, 65 N.E. 865 (1902). See also *Bruni v. Tatsumi,* 46 Ohio St. 2d 127, 129, 346 N.E. 2d 673, 676 (1976).

(Author's note: the "locality" rule no longer pertains in most jurisdictions.)

Statute of Limitations

Declaring that no suit shall be maintained unless brought within a specified time after the right accured.

Strict Liability

A concept applied by the courts in product liability cases in which a seller is liable for any and all defective or hazardous products which unduly threaten a consumer's personal safety.

Substantial Evidence

Evidence which a reasoning mind would accept as sufficient to support a particular conclusion and consists of more than a mere scintilla of evidence but may be somewhat less than a preponderance.

Marker v. Finch, 322 F. Supp. 905, 910 (D. Del. 1971).

Tort

A private or civil wrong or injury, other than breach of contract, for which the court will provide a remedy in the form of an action for damages. There must always be a violation of some duty owing to the plaintiff. The elements of every tort action are existence of a legal duty from the defendant to the plaintiff, breach of duty, and damage as a proximate result.

Joseph v. Hustad Corp., 454 P. 2d 916, 918 (Mont. 1969).

Vicarious Liability

Indirect legal responsibility, e.g., employer for employee or principal for agent.

Weight of Evidence

The balance or preponderance of evidence; the inclination of the greater amount of credible evidence offered in a trial to support one side of the issue rather than the other. Weight depends on its effect in including belief.

Index